CONTENTS

ACKNOWLEDGEMENTS

Panos wishes to acknowledge the help given by many individuals and organisations across the world in preparing this publication. Many people quoted in the text gave background information or reviewed early drafts of the text; in particular, thanks must be given to Calle Almedal and Shivananda Khan. Among those not named in the text but who also assisted were Lucy Atkin, Gloria Coe, Tim France, Peter Gordon, Judith Helzner, Stuart Kingma, Sue Lucas, Rubén Mayorga, Chandra Mouli, Marjorie Muecke, Richard Parker, Marty Radlett, Matthew Roberts, Melissa Root, Marcela Sánchez-Bender, Bernhard Schwartlander, Veriano Terto and John Watson; we apologise to those whose names have been inadvertently omitted.

Jonathan Mann continued a tradition of ten years helping Panos by suggesting individuals to contact for research; this book is dedicated to his work and memory.

PREFACE

At night in a small village, a man taps his wife's shoulder. Aware of the children sleeping beside them, she silently pulls up her clothing and lets him enter her.

A hundred miles away in a comfortable city apartment, a young woman and her husband make love affectionately.

In a park in the centre of the city, two married men make eye contact. One drops to his knees as the other exposes himself.

Not far away, a woman in her twenties greets her eighth client of the evening, a man 30 years older.

The next afternoon, a teenage girl goes to bed with the businessman who pays for her education.

In the bush, a man in his early twenties molests his seven-year-old nephew. Later that day, his younger brother will persuade his girlfriend to surrender her virginity to him.

That evening in a seaport, an unemployed man returns home drunk and rapes his wife.

Nearby, a young man takes an old syringe, siphons up a bubbling brown paste, injects half into himself and passes the syringe to his friend.

Next door, two men who have known each other for years make love.

A few blocks away, a man negotiates the price of sexual services with a man in woman's clothing.

In the suburbs, a woman in her sixties entices her husband to bed.

The settings and characters may change, but the scenes are universal. The village could be in India, Mali or Bolivia. The apartment might be in Vancouver, Nairobi or Buenos Aires. The park could be in the same city, or in Dhaka, Dakar or Rio de Janeiro. The tourist might be European or North American, Asian, African or Middle Eastern. Such sexual and drug-injecting activity can be found on every continent, in almost every country, irrespective of law, religion or custom. In each case, if one partner has HIV - the virus which causes AIDS - it may be passed to the other, and in each case transmission could be prevented.

Each scene includes a man because without men there would be no AIDS epidemic. Men are involved in almost every case of sexual transmission; perhaps one in every 10 cases is the result of transmission solely between men. Four of every five drug injectors are men. With more sexual and drug-taking partners than women, men have more opportunity to transmit HIV. More often than not, it is men who determine whether sex takes place and whether a condom is used. In general, women are more liable to contract HIV without passing it on, men more liable both to contract and transmit the virus to others.

Men and women both fall sick and die from AIDS, but in many ways men are less affected by the disease. Worldwide, women are contracting HIV at a faster rate than men. Women with the virus may pass it to their future children. At home and in hospital, women assume greater responsibility for caring for the sick.

Not every man is likely to transmit HIV to others. Perhaps no more than a quarter of men endanger themselves and their female or male partners in this way. Yet that one in four represents hundreds of millions of men who, it appears, regularly act without thought and leave women to deal with the consequences of their actions.

Those responsible for the AIDS epidemic are also at risk. A man cannot transmit HIV to others unless he contracts it first himself; the same act - unprotected sexual intercourse or drug injection without sterilisation - jeopardises himself as much as his partner. Why do some men regularly risk their own lives, the lives of their loved ones and the lives of acquaintances and strangers? Can men be persuaded to change their behaviour?

This book is divided into two sections. The first examines the relationship between men's actions and AIDS around the world, the impact of those actions on men and women and initiatives designed to help men protect themselves and their partners. The second section, written by journalists from 11 countries in the Americas, Africa, Asia and Eastern Europe, illustrates many different aspects of that relationship - from machismo in Mexico to drug injection in Russia, from men in prison in Brazil to men living with HIV in Thailand, from men as fathers in the Ivory Coast to men who have sex with men in Kenya.

The country reports were commissioned with two goals in mind. The first was to put a human face on the many different relationships between men and women and between men and men which lie behind the global AIDS epidemic. The second was to stimulate discussion on the issue, particularly within the countries in which the reports were commissioned. In addition to global distribution of this book, one or more chapters are being published in each of the 11 countries; both there and elsewhere, those who work on AIDS, health, gender issues and social justice are encouraged to contribute to the ongoing debate on the question of men and HIV.

Men undoubtedly take risks in relation to HIV. Whether or not they should also take responsibility for transmission of the virus, and how they can do so, are questions that cannot be resolved easily. If this book provides some insights that allow a greater understanding of the issue, it will have achieved its purpose.

INTRODUCTION
ARE MEN TO BLAME?

"The HIV epidemic is driven by men," says Calle Almedal, a senior official with the Joint United Nations AIDS Programme (UNAIDS). His opinion is shared by other AIDS experts and is confirmed by statistical analysis of the disease. Worldwide, women* may be more affected by the consequences of HIV/AIDS, but it is the sexual and drug-taking behaviour of a large minority of men which enables the virus to spread.

Men's behaviour threatens women. More men than women are HIV-positive - living with the virus - but the social and physical factors underlying the epidemic mean that this ratio will almost certainly be reversed in the next decade. Not only will most women with the virus fall ill with AIDS, but many will pass the virus to their newborn children and most will also take on the burden of caring for other family members with the disease.

In recognition of their vulnerability, women have been the target of many AIDS prevention programmes. The programmes raise awareness of HIV and enable some women to protect themselves through condoms or abstinence from sex, but most have little impact on the overall course of the epidemic. Men usually decide whether women can protect themselves and men are more likely than women to transmit the virus to others, including other

---

* Unless otherwise specified, references to 'men' and 'women' in this book include boys and girls who have reached sexual maturity.

men. In short, men determine the path of the disease. Only prevention programmes that directly address men's sexual and drug-taking behaviour can significantly reduce the rate at which the global HIV/AIDS epidemic spreads.

Vulnerability and risk

Women are vulnerable to HIV; men are at risk. That generalisation reflects the different circumstances in which both sexes contract the disease. Most women are vulnerable because they have limited opportunity to protect themselves; many men are at risk because they refuse to do so - often deliberately, it seems.

Specific patterns of sexual behaviour underlie women's vulnerability. Many (perhaps most) adults and teenagers are not at risk of contracting HIV, either because they are sexually abstinent or because they are faithful to partners who are faithful to them. For others, the risk varies. Men are more likely to have two or more concurrent or consecutive partners and are therefore at greater risk both of contracting the virus and passing it on; women are more likely to be faithful to men from whom they contract HIV and less likely to pass it on.

Women's vulnerability is heightened by other factors. Men's refusal to use condoms or to stop relations with other partners denies women opportunities to protect themselves. HIV passes more easily from men to women than vice versa. Other sexually transmitted infections (STIs, often known as STDs) make it easier to transmit HIV; not only are women more liable to contract such infections but they are less likely to be aware of the fact and are less likely to seek treatment. Some men have sex with other men, and the relative ease of HIV transmission between men increases the risk to their female partners. Patterns of drug injection - men are more likely to share needles with several partners while women are more likely to share only with one man - similarly increase men's risk and women's vulnerability.

Underlying all these considerations are a range of social and economic factors which restrict women's freedom to control their own lives, particularly their sexual lives. Poverty, illiteracy and traditional customs often combine to prevent women either from knowing what they must do to protect themselves or, if they know, from taking action to do so.

Some men and adolescent boys are also vulnerable. Those who are younger, poorer or physically or psychologically weaker are liable to contract HIV from other men through sex or shared drug-injecting equipment. Those who take the recipient role in anal intercourse are especially vulnerable. Transvestites and transsexuals and pre-adolescent children may also be compelled by force or circumstance into situations where they contract HIV from men.

Responsibility and blame

Even when they are aware of the risk of contracting and transmitting HIV, many men fail to protect themselves and their partners. This failure leads some commentators to consider men responsible, or even to blame, for the HIV/AIDS epidemic. Others argue that the responsibility for transmitting HIV lies less with individual men or with men as a group than with widely accepted concepts of masculinity that underpin the behaviour of millions of men across the globe.

Throughout the short history of AIDS, different groups have been blamed for the disease: men who have sex with men in the United States, Africans in Eastern Europe, women sex workers in many countries. Blame may provide a short-term emotional outlet, but it usually stems from ignorance or prejudice and frequently diverts attention from measures that would reduce the impact and extent of the disease. Blaming men would likely have the same negative effect.

While a minority of men with more than one sexual or drug-injecting partner can be depicted as 'responsible' for the spread of HIV, that does not mean they intentionally pass on the virus.

Cases where individuals deliberately transmit HIV to others are rare and usually the result of mental disturbance or lack of understanding of the risks. Ignorance, lack of access to condoms and lack of skill in negotiating protection also play a part.

Above all, many if not most men who fail to protect themselves and their partners do so less from conscious choice than because that is how men are expected to behave. Most boys grow up believing, implicitly or explicitly, that their identity as men, and therefore as individuals, is defined by their sexual prowess. Attitudes towards sex are in a state of flux almost everywhere, but in many societies men are still expected to have frequent intercourse with their wives or regular partners and occasional or regular intercourse with casual partners. Women are expected to accede to men's demands, abstinence is seen as harmful, and condoms are seen as unmasculine or as restricting a man's pleasure. As long as men - and women - are influenced by such concepts of masculinity, HIV will continue to spread.

The wrong target?

Many imaginative AIDS prevention programmes have been targeted at women, partly out of recognition of their vulnerability and partly from an assumption that, once convinced of the need to use condoms, women would be able to persuade their partners to do so. Yet although many women can and do control their sexual lives, a considerably greater number find it difficult to persuade their male partners to use a condom or to abstain from sex with other women. A large number of others refuse to challenge their partners for fear of a violent reaction.

Of those women who have managed to protect themselves, it is only sex workers, or other women with more than one sexual partner, whose changed behaviour significantly reduces the rate at which HIV spreads. In epidemiological terms, this means that many prevention programmes have addressed the wrong target. Persuading 10 men with several partners to use condoms, sterilise needles or have fewer partners has a far greater impact on the epidemic than enabling 1,000 women to protect themselves from their only partner. The 10 men are at the beginning of a chain of infection; the 1,000 women are its last link.

This does not mean abandoning prevention programmes for women whose only risk is their partner; everyone who might contract HIV should be informed of their vulnerability and of steps they can take to protect themselves. It is, however, precisely to assist women to protect themselves that men must also be a focus for prevention activities.

Confronting the challenge

Prevention programmes that succeed in changing men's behaviour protect both the men and their partners: regular and casual partners of either sex, sex workers and drug injectors. Such prevention programmes affect the wider course of the AIDS epidemic, as can be seen in countries as diverse as Australia, Senegal, Thailand, the United Kingdom and Uganda, where behaviour change by large numbers of men - and to a lesser extent by women - has resulted in either static or falling HIV transmission rates.

Apparent success in a few countries does not mean that changing men's behaviour is easy. Furthermore, not all men behave alike. Many men either are not at risk or consistently protect themselves and others against transmission. Worldwide, at any one time perhaps only one man in four is liable to contract or transmit HIV.

Yet even if relatively few are responsible for the spread of HIV, all men should take responsibility for their sexual behaviour. A first step in that direction is to encourage greater understanding of the relationship between men, HIV/AIDS and the societies in which both men and women live. As *AIDS and Men* attempts to show, the physical, social and psychological factors which lead men to place themselves and others at risk allow no single, easy solution.

PART ONE

MEN, SEX AND HIV

Epidemics such as measles, cholera and malaria do not spread evenly through a population: who contracts an infection and how quickly it moves between individuals depend on factors which vary from community to community and from disease to disease. So it is not surprising that the profile of HIV/AIDS differs between and even within countries. Nevertheless, whichever group is involved – whether drug injectors, young women, or men who have sex with men – each epidemic is directly attributable to the sexual and drug-injecting behaviour of a significant minority of men.

Although HIV is primarily spread through sex, not everyone who is sexually active is liable to contract it. Men appear to be at greater risk because, on average, they have more partners than women; in fact, greater numbers of women are vulnerable – both the relatively small number who have many sexual partners and the far greater number who may contract the virus from unfaithful male partners. Furthermore, women's vulnerability is heightened by physical factors which make it easier for men to pass HIV to women than vice versa.

Casual affairs

Even allowing for people's tendency to under- or over-estimate their sexual contacts, in every society surveyed, men appear to have more sexual partners than women. In any 12-month period, most teenagers and adults are

The Joy of Sex?

Successful HIV prevention depends on persuading millions of men and women to adopt specific forms of sexual behaviour. The task is made more difficult by the fact that sex is only partly subject to rational decision-making. Not only are biological factors such as erection, ejaculation, the production of vaginal fluid and orgasm not under our conscious control, but they are strongly influenced by social and psychological imperatives.

Thus young men are often pressured into sex by the need to 'prove themselves', while young women submit to the demands of their suitors, and some women and men are forced to exchange sex for food and shelter. A woman may have sex with her husband one night from desire, another night in return for a favour she wants from him and a third night because he demands it. A sex worker has intercourse with a client for money and with a long-term partner for pleasure and intimacy. A man who has sex with his wife to father children has very different motives when he establishes power over another man by raping him.

In summary, as Rwandan commentator Damien Rwegera points out, sex involves "the pursuit of pleasure, desire for intimacy, expression of love, definition of self, procreation, domination, violence or any combination of the above. How people relate sexually may be linked to self-esteem, self-respect, respect for others, hope, joy and pain. In different contexts, sex is viewed as a commodity, a right or a biological imperative" [4].

Millions of couples find sexual fulfilment; millions more are inhibited by such factors as lack of privacy, ignorance or taboos that prevent the discussion of topics as simple as physical discomfort or as important as the wish to use a condom. This means that each year millions of people die from AIDS, syphilis and other consequences of sexual ignorance.

Because men usually have greater control over intercourse than their female partners, they are more likely to derive satisfaction from sex. In contrast, many women across the world would echo this comment from India: "I do not know who makes love to me. My husband tells me he wants sex. I lie back, pull my sari over my head and wait. I suppose he is the one who enters me, but it could be any man" [5].

Men's satisfaction, however, may be as much from achieving the act itself as from any intrinsic pleasure. Shivananda Khan, who works in AIDS prevention in South Asia, says that sexual activity for most poor men in the region is motivated "less by desire than by discharge; in such circumstances even the gender of the partner is less important than the opportunity she or he offers for discharge." I.S. Gilada of the Indian Health Organisation confirms this by reporting that many clients of sex workers in Mumbai (Bombay) feel no sense of elation after the act, although this may be related to a widespread sense among men of anticlimax after sex, irrespective of the circumstances. ■

abstinent or faithful to their current sexual partner, but a large minority of men and a small minority of women have concurrent (overlapping) sexual relationships. Furthermore, over a lifetime men have considerably more partners than women, which means they have more opportunity to contract and pass on HIV.

In 1995 the World Health Organization (WHO) published the results of a survey into sexual behaviour in 18 countries. In every country more men than women admitted to casual partners in the preceding 12 months, from four percent in Sri Lanka (compared to three percent of women), through 38 percent in Guinea Bissau (19 percent of women) to 45 percent (10 percent of women) in Rio de Janeiro, Brazil [1]. In the late 1980s, 70 percent of women interviewed in Costa Rica claimed to have had only one sexual partner, compared to nine percent of men; while 99 percent of the women interviewed said they had had no more than five partners in their lifetime, 55 percent of the men claimed six or more [2]. The British National Survey of Sexual Attitudes and Lifestyles, published in 1994, found that whereas 24 percent of men claimed 10 or more women partners in their lifetime, only seven percent of women claimed the same number of male partners [3].

While most men have sex only with women, sex between men occurs in every society, even where it is highly taboo; three to 16 percent of men report having sex with other men. This is explored in more detail later in the book. Sex also occurs between women, but HIV is seldom transmitted in such circumstances.

Driving the epidemic

In epidemiological terms, there are three groups of people: those at little or no risk of contracting HIV, those at risk of contracting the virus but unlikely to transmit it to others, and those who are liable both to contract and transmit the virus. The last group, sometimes defined as the 'core group', drives the epidemic. It may consist of men and women or only of sexually active or drug-injecting men, but, whatever its focus and size, no core group can exist without men [6].

Those at little or no risk include men and women who have never had sex; who are currently abstinent; who consistently practise 'safer sex' (with condoms or without penetration); and those who are in a relationship in which both partners are HIV-negative and faithful to each other. Those who may contract the virus but are unlikely to transmit it to others are individuals who are faithful to their partner but whose partner either contracted HIV in a previous relationship or is unfaithful and has unprotected sex with others. Those who are liable to transmit HIV include all individuals who have unprotected sex with more than one partner. (Men and women in polygamous relationships are not at risk if all partners are faithful to the relationship and no partner contracted HIV before the relationship began.)

The WHO statistics quoted above suggest that (a) there are more women than men in the first group (at little or no risk) because men are more likely to have casual sex and women are more likely to be abstinent; (b) there are more women than men in the second group (at risk of contracting

HIV), because women are more likely to be faithful to partners who are not; and (c) there are more men than women in the third group (the 'core group', liable to transmit HIV to others) because more men have casual partners [7].

The size of the core group determines the likely extent of the epidemic in a community. Where the core group is a small proportion of the population, the epidemic is likely to be restricted, since even if the number of those at risk of contracting but not transmitting HIV is larger than the core, the virus will not go beyond that second group. In Australia, for example, the epidemic is restricted because the core (in this case, men who have sex with many men) is small. However, where many people have unprotected sex with more than one partner, the concept of a core group is less meaningful and a greater proportion of the population may contract the infection. In parts of sub-Saharan Africa, for example, one in four adults is HIV-positive.

The more partners with whom an individual has unprotected sex, the greater the likelihood of transmitting the virus to others. One study reports truck drivers in India visiting between 50 and 100 sex workers a year [8]. A survey in Harare, Zimbabwe, reports that some men visit sex workers an average of 7.4 times a month [9]; even if, as claimed, condoms are used on half of these occasions, that still means each has 40 unprotected acts of intercourse with different partners a year – hence 40 opportunities to contract or transmit HIV. One survey of gay men's lifestyles in New York in the late 1970s showed that respondents had an average of 41 partners a year, a figure that explains the rapid diffusion of the virus in that community in the period immediately before people became aware of the disease [10].

Some women have many sex partners; those who are unable or unwilling to use condoms – and therefore who risk contracting and transmitting HIV – form part of the core group. However, their numbers are small in comparison to men. A far greater number of women are at risk because they are faithful to partners who are not faithful to them [11]. The impact of men's sexual behaviour on women can be seen in places such as Kigali, Rwanda, where women with no other risk factor except their long-term partner form the largest proportion of women with HIV or AIDS [12].

Physical factors

The risk of contracting HIV in any one act of intercourse or shared injection in which one partner has the virus cannot be calculated. Women's social vulnerability to HIV – the fact that women are likely to have male partners who do not protect themselves from the virus – is heightened by a range of physical factors which make it easier for a man to transmit HIV to a woman than vice versa. Some men are also made more vulnerable by these factors.

vaginal intercourse

Apart from solitary masturbation, vaginal intercourse is probably the most widely practised sexual act. In the absence of other factors, a man with HIV probably has a one in 500 chance of passing the virus to his partner in a single act of unprotected vaginal intercourse. The odds of woman-to-man transmission in the same circumstances are about one in 1,000 [13].

anal intercourse

HIV transmission through unprotected anal intercourse occurs through the mucous membrane of the rectum or minute ruptures to the rectum and penis; the risk of transmission for the recipient partner is much higher than for unprotected vaginal intercourse [14]. Anal intercourse is practised between men and between men and women. It has been reported at least once by 16 percent of middle-class married women surveyed in India [15], 17 percent of adolescent girls surveyed in Zambia [16] and 19 percent of college women surveyed in North America [17]. It has been argued that the extent of anal intercourse between men is underestimated in many countries and this may distort analysis of the epidemic [18]. The same may be true for anal intercourse between men and women.

other sexually-transmitted infections

Each year there are an estimated 333 million new cases of sexually transmitted infection (STI) [19]. STIs which cause ulcers or lesions allow HIV to enter the bloodstream directly, multiplying the risk of infection up to sevenfold [20]. Like HIV, most STIs are transmitted more easily from men to women than vice versa.

Men are usually aware of discharge or visible lesions in the penis and may therefore seek treatment. They are less likely to be aware of infections in the anus and, in many countries, doctors will neither look for nor treat anal infections. Some infections contracted anally, such as syphilis, can be transmitted both anally and through blood and semen.

Women are less likely to seek treatment for sexually transmitted infections, because lesions are usually internal and discharge may be confused with period flow or vaginal fluid; because many cultures discourage women from learning about STIs; or because they may not be able to afford treatment. In short, other sexually transmitted infections are an additional factor placing women, and men who practise recipient anal intercourse, at significantly greater risk of contracting HIV.

other factors in vaginal intercourse

Women's increased susceptibility through vaginal intercourse can be worsened by other factors. Those under

20 are more vulnerable than those who are older because their relatively immature genital tract has fewer layers of mucous membrane and is thus more liable to infection. Genital mutilation (also known as female circumcision) increases the risk if it leads to bleeding during intercourse [21], while practices such as dry sex (see the report from Tanzania below) may also increase the likelihood of male-to-female transmission [22].

viral load

Viral load measures the amount of HIV in the blood. This is very high during the first few months after an individual contracts the virus [23]. Because a man is more likely than a woman to have sex with another partner soon after contracting HIV, and because the viral load rises in seminal but not vaginal fluid [24], men are more likely to transmit the virus to others during this period. The rapid spread of HIV in some communities, such as men who have sex with men in the United States in the 1970s-1980s, and throughout Thailand in the 1980s, has been attributed to many people having other sexual partners soon after contracting the virus.

drug injection

HIV transmission occurs during drug injection when infected blood from one injector is injected into a second and subsequent injectors through shared equipment. The risk of transmission through shared equipment is believed to be at least 1 in 200 [25], but is likely to be considerably greater if viral load is high. Not only are 80 percent of drug injectors estimated to be men, but the fact that men are more likely to share needles* with other men, while women are more likely to share only with their male partner, means that transmission between men and from

* 'Needle' refers to all parts of the manufactured or makeshift syringe where blood may mingle with the substance to be injected.

men to women is more common than from women to men. This is discussed later in the book.

male circumcision [26]

Some studies suggest that men who are not circumcised are at greater risk of contracting and transmitting HIV in unprotected sex [27].

oral intercourse

The extent to which fellatio (mouth-penis contact) and cunnilingus (mouth-vagina contact) are practised differs from culture to culture. No studies have proven any risk attached to cunnilingus. Similarly, no study has shown that a man is at risk from inserting his penis into the mouth of a person with HIV. There is some risk to a woman or a man who takes into their mouth the penis of a man with HIV; the seriousness of the risk is uncertain, although it is believed to be considerably lower than from vaginal sex. Sores or lesions in the mouth or on the penis increase the risk of contracting HIV, as does ejaculation.

viral subtype

It has been suggested that two strains of HIV (sub-types C and E) are more easily transmitted via the vagina, which may partially explain infection among men and women in sub-Saharan Africa and South-East Asia, where these sub-types are predominant [28]. However, at least one study has found no correlation between sub-type and means of transmission [29].

Emerging epidemics

The impact of these factors varies, with the result that the global HIV/AIDS epidemic is best described as a series of epidemics focusing on different, sometimes small, sometimes diffuse core groups. Core groups may be geographically and

Till Condom Come

Only abstinence guarantees that HIV transmission will not occur, but consistent 'safer sex' practices - use of condoms and non-penetrative sex - reduce transmission to near-insignificant levels. One study in Haiti showed that couples who consistently used male condoms had one seventh of the HIV transmission rate of those who did not [32], while use of male condoms has been credited with reductions in HIV transmission rates throughout Thailand [33].

As discussed in the next chapter, many men are unlikely to regard abstinence or non-penetrative sex as serious options. However, the male condom is not always considered easy to use, and lack of familiarity and reluctance to discuss its use contribute to high failure rates. In some studies, condoms have broken or slipped off in up to five out of 100 acts of vaginal intercourse where at least some of the men had little experience with condoms [34].

This perception of failure, together with implied infidelity and other factors described below, lie behind many men's refusal to use condoms. Many women are reluctant to suggest them for fear of the reaction the request might provoke. As a South African research team comments, "Women commonly find themselves wholly unable to negotiate the timing of sex and the conditions under which it occurs. Many of them feel powerless even to protect themselves against pregnancy. Condom use is far from being a possibility in their lives" [35].

The female condom has some advantages over the male version, including women's greater control over its use and the fact that it does not cling to the penis. Surveys in several countries show that couples generally welcome it, although some find it inconvenient and noisy. The female condom is increasingly available in the developing world, but its cost remains much higher than that of the male version (about US$1.00 each compared to US$0.05, although tests suggest that the female condom can be reused [36]) and women still have to negotiate its use.

Stronger male condoms and the female version can also be used for anal sex between men [37] and between men and women. Prevention campaigns advise condoms and lubricants for anal sex between men but a range of factors, including unavailability, high cost or embarrassment, prevent many men from obtaining them.

Meanwhile, failure to address the fact that men practise anal sex with women may increase the risk of HIV transmission. Daniel Halperin, a prevention expert who has worked in the US and Brazil, claims that "nearly all campaigns, at least implicitly, equate intercourse between men and women with vaginal sex" [38]. As a result, Halperin says, condoms are used less frequently for anal sex between men and women than for vaginal sex. ■

socially restricted, such as drug injectors in one city or soldiers from one barracks, but they can also cross boundaries. Thus there is one epidemic among sexually active men and women in eastern Africa, another among injecting drug users and their partners in Russia, and a third among men who have sex with men in the United Kingdom. These epidemics may be discrete or overlap. In New York, for example, where men who have sex with men comprise one epidemic and injecting drug users comprise another, some men belong to both groups. There may also be disagreement over the profile of an epidemic. Opinion differs, for instance, as to whether the primary epidemic in India is between men and women or whether there is a 'hidden' epidemic driven by sex between men.

If a core group transmits HIV to enough partners with a different pattern of behaviour, another epidemic may emerge. There has been much debate in the industrialised world as to whether the primary epidemics of drug injection and sex between men in countries such as Italy and the United States will transmit the infection to enough other people to create an epidemic driven by sex between men and women. So far, it appears that the level of unprotected sexual activity between men and women in these countries has not been high enough for a new epidemic to emerge [30].

This does not mean that countries which have been spared extensive epidemics will avoid them in the future. Patterns of behaviour can change significantly in a relatively short time. It has been argued that a sudden increase in the rate of anal intercourse between men in North America allowed the virus to spread rapidly in that population in the 1970s [31]; it is possible that decolonisation, urbanisation and migration led to weakened family and community ties in parts of sub-Saharan Africa, leading to changes in sexual behaviour which allowed the virus to spread rapidly in the 1980s. As described in a later chapter, the fashion for injecting drugs has led to an explosion of HIV infection among young men in Russia in the 1990s. Similar changes may occur in other countries in the future.

One in four

This chapter can provide only a simple analysis of the complexity of the global AIDS epidemic [39]. Most men do not place themselves or their partners at risk of contracting HIV. Indeed, if the WHO statistics quoted elsewhere are averaged out, perhaps no more than one in three or one in four men worldwide is sexually active with more than one partner or shares injecting equipment with others. But that figure is high enough to maintain a localised or nationwide AIDS epidemic in almost every country.

Preventing HIV transmission among the core group has a significantly greater impact on the epidemic than preventing transmission among the general population. One study suggests that preventing 100 cases of HIV in the non-core population prevents an additional 180 cases in the following 10 years, while preventing 100 cases in the core population prevents almost 10 times that number [40]. It has therefore been argued that "the principles of public economics and epidemiology are ... that governments should give high priority to the prevention of infection among people most likely to contract and spread HIV" [41].

This approach is epidemiologically sound but can be problematic on other grounds. Core groups are not static and may comprise a considerable proportion of the population.

Sex workers may be active for only two or three years, men with many sexual partners may settle down after marriage or return to such behaviour if the marriage breaks down, and millions of young people become sexually active each year.

In some cases groups at risk, such as the military, can be identified and targeted by specific programmes devised to encourage them to change their behaviour. In other cases there are ethical problems and technical difficulties in singling out groups such as drug injectors or men who have sex with men. Inappropriate action, such as arrest or refusal to supply sterile equipment, may restrict their human rights and lead to further dissemination of the virus as those who are affected 'go underground'. Indeed, criminalising or stigmatising HIV-related behaviour seldom leads to reduced transmission. Illegal drug injection continues despite determined efforts to stamp it out, while female and male prostitution and semi-public sexual activities between men are common in many countries where such activities are illegal.

Whatever approach is adopted to reduce transmission, it must take into account the causes of people's behaviour, particularly the behaviour of those men whose practices drive the epidemic. The following chapters examine two key issues underlying the spread of HIV: why do a minority of men consistently endanger themselves and others, and how can we persuade those men to change their behaviour?

What Makes a Man?

Why do a considerable minority of men persist in placing themselves and their partners at risk? If we can answer that question, we will be closer to devising strategies for those men and thereby reducing the overall rate at which HIV and other diseases spread.

In every society, men's conduct is determined at least in part by widely held perceptions as to how men should behave – perceptions shared by women as much as men. Men are expected to be physically and emotionally strong, to take risks and to have frequent sexual intercourse, often with more than one partner. These deeply rooted expectations lead many men to insist on sex when their partners do not want it, to consider condoms unmanly and to see drug injection as illicit, dangerous and therefore attractive.

Masculinity brings with it privileges and, in many societies, freedoms denied to most women. Such privileges, however, impose burdens, with many men having sex and refusing condoms because they are conditioned to do so rather than because they want to. Furthermore, subconsciously, some men resent the obligations imposed on them; that resentment is often manifested in anger and violence towards women and other men.

It is, however, irrelevant whether a man places himself, his partners and his future children at risk because he welcomes the privileges offered by his masculine status, or whether he is driven to do so from fear of losing that status. The problem, in terms of HIV/AIDS prevention, is less the attitudes of individual men than those of the societies in which they live – attitudes which lie at the heart of the epidemic.

Men and women

That men and women behave differently is not in doubt, but why they do so is a debate that may not be resolved for generations. In the West, one strand of research sees some differences in behaviour between the sexes, such as men's tendency to have more sexual partners, as biologically determined [1], while others are convinced all differences are culturally induced [2]. The debate is further complicated by the fact that some individuals are born with physical or chromosomal differences from the majority of men and women, while others who are physically or chromosomally all male or all female identify themselves strongly as the opposite gender or as an intergender.

Broadly speaking, the biological argument claims that because a woman bears and suckles children, she needs only one sexual partner, who will be a father to her children and will protect and nourish her and those children; because a man (until the advent of DNA testing) could not be sure that he was the father of his partner's children, he seeks many sexual partners to increase the chances that at least one of them will give birth to his child. The cultural argument is that all relationships between the sexes, including men's greater wealth, status and political power, reflect no more than the control over women derived from men's greater physical strength.

Even if masculinity is biologically determined, it is interpreted differently in different cultures. "The factors that influence a man's behaviours in a traditional African community will in some ways differ and in some ways potentially be very similar to those that influence an urban

European or Asian man" [3]. Shivananda Khan of the Naz Foundation, a non-governmental organisation (NGO) working in South Asia, says that in India malehood and femalehood are partly defined by family, community and social duties. A man might be extremely effeminate in Western eyes, but he is seen as manly if he has fulfilled his community duties as a married man with sons. A single man, even if extremely masculine in a Western sense, is defined as not-yet-a-man [4]. This male status (*sandh* in Hindi) – unmarried, probably fun-loving and slightly irresponsible – is recognised across the globe, from the *bujang* of Indonesia to the Bangladeshi *zubok*, the Italian *ragazzo* and the Brazilian *rapaz*.

Whatever the roots of masculinity, the word is difficult to define, not only because each society views men differently, but because 'masculinity' combines observations as to how men *do* behave and opinions as to how they *should* behave. Furthermore, ideas of masculinity are changing rapidly in many societies, particularly among the middle classes, and behaviour that was accepted in men a generation or more ago is often rejected today.

Masculinity and virility

Irrespective of its origins, some aspects of masculinity appear to be common to cultures in which most of the world's population live. Details may differ, but men are expected to be strong and daring, to be the primary provider of their families' food and shelter and to defend themselves, their families and their societies from aggressors. Traditionally, it is men rather than women who take risks, whether fighting battles, climbing mountains, racing cars or breaking the law.

The sexual component of masculinity is virility, defined by a man's ability to penetrate. In many societies, even where prevailing mores exhort them to abstain from sex before marriage, young men are expected to prove their sexual prowess. In some cultures, fathers 'initiate' their sons by taking them to prostitutes [5]; in many cultures young men are expected to coerce their girlfriends into intercourse. As described elsewhere in this book, in Uganda a generation ago, "while there was always uproar if an unmarried girl became pregnant, boys were always encouraged by their peers and fathers to prove they were not impotent."

To be a boy or man does not automatically mean being masculine. Some individuals who are born anatomically and/or chromosomally male reject many or all attributes of masculinity and adopt culturally recognised roles as effeminate men or 'non-men'. Effeminacy is usually associated with being penetrated by other men, such as the *cabro* or *marica* in Peru or the *khoti* in South Asia. Those who completely reject masculinity, including *travestis* in Brazil and *hijras* in India, often modify their bodies to fit their chosen status, taking hormones to develop breasts or undergoing operations, which may be extremely crude, to lose their genitalia.

Out of control

Many people believe that a man's need for sex is beyond his control, with young men in particular suffering physical and mental damage if intercourse is denied. Thais of both sexes say men "have strong sexual desire and need some outlet" [6]. South African miners claim that regular intercourse is essential for a man's good health [7], and in Indian society "it is considered natural for men to be 'lustful'" [8]. This viewpoint appears universal. One US commentator refers to the common notion that "males, straight or gay, are at the mercy of biological forces beyond their control, forces that impel us to seek as many partners as possible" [9]. An Australian commentator claims that men's sexual behaviour is subconsciously driven by their simultaneous desire for, and fear of, loss of control [10].

Sex and Rape

Interpretations of sex vary both within and across cultures. Some Western commentators argue that men define sex as vaginal or anal penetration while women define it less as physical activity than as emotional bonding. Asian researchers point out that some forms of behaviour defined as sex in the West have little or no sexual connotations in their country [13].

For some commentators penetration represents domination, and it is no coincidence that in almost every language the vulgarism 'to fuck' also means to defeat or humiliate; from this perspective, all penetration is rape because all intercourse is domination. Others argue that a range of attitudes, actions and emotions lie behind intercourse and there is no imbalance of power if the recipient partner (woman or man) wishes to be penetrated.

Many men do not consider sex a consensual activity. Wives are often beaten for refusing to submit to their husbands and many women are at risk outside the home. South Africa sees an estimated 1.3 million rapes a year [14] – one for every nine sexually active men. It is the powerless who are usually the victims. One study of six American and Asian countries disclosed that between 13 and 29 percent of rape and sexual assault victims were aged under 10, and between 36 and 62 percent were under 15. The same study reported that 60 percent of women in the United States who first had sex before the age of 15 described it as involuntary, while in Barbados one in three young men and women report having been sexually abused in childhood or adolescence [15]. ■

Polygynous societies (where a man may have more than one wife*) formalise the belief that men cannot be sexually restricted to one woman. Polygyny is authorised by religion and law in Islamic countries and sanctioned by social attitudes in parts of the Caribbean or Africa, where some men live with their wives while maintaining separate households for their other children and the mothers of

* Polyandry, which is rare, refers to women with more than one husband. Polygamy refers to both polygyny and polyandry.

those children. Polygyny is often supported by women as much as men. Marie-Louise Ndala Musuamba of the (then) Zairean Network on Ethics, Law and HIV comments: "A mother often teaches her son that he will become the husband of several wives and, as such, their chief. This mentality has encouraged men to seek out multiple sexual partners and has even influenced the law, which condemns men's acts of adultery only if they assume an insulting character" [11].

Virility does not always insist that men have sex only with women; in some cultures a man who penetrates other men is still seen as virile. For a man to be penetrated, however, whether voluntarily or through force, almost always stigmatises him as effeminate. In Mexico, where homosexuality is equated with femaleness, penetrating other men "is not considered homosexual … Indeed, having sex in this way with other men may in fact reaffirm his masculinity as the penetrator of others. The opposite is true for the man who allows himself to be penetrated. He is the only one likely to be seen as homosexual" [12]. In a few societies, however, such as the Keraki of New Guinea, boys become men through receptive anal intercourse.

Fragile men

Masculinity is a very public trait, which on the one hand offers power and privilege but on the other hand imposes a role model which not all men welcome. Indeed, many live in conscious or subconscious fear that they do not live up to masculine ideals. As one Western commentator writes, "Most studies show masculinity as rather fragile, provisional, something to be won and then defended, something under constant threat of loss" [16].

Men are encouraged to 'be a man' by other men and ridicule is the reward for those who fail. Richard, a 17-year-old Ugandan, spent time with other young men who "tried to persuade me to do what they were doing by sending me different girls." Uncomfortable with the pressure and unable to initiate conversation and sexual intercourse, he was teased and mocked by the group: "'Richard, you seem to be impotent – were you castrated?' To sum it up, they deserted me on those grounds" [17].

Men's insecurity and fears manifest themselves in different ways. Fear that they cannot 'perform' with their wives causes some Zimbabwean men to resort to herbs to maintain an erection [18]. A similar fear may lie behind much of the demand in the United States for the impotence cure Viagra. Fear of losing their authority makes many male political and religious leaders hostile to educational and economic advances for women. Fear of ridicule, of being seen as 'less than a man', lies behind much of the violence men inflict on strangers or their wives [19].

"Boys and men are pushed to be braver and more aggressive when they feel fear. In men, fear is transformed into aggression and in women, submission," says one commentator [20]. "Boys are not taught survival skills the way girls are," says Patricia Burke of the Jamaican National AIDS Committee. "In the absence of this training, they depend heavily on the women in their lives but they are unhappy about it. They have internalised the ideology of male dominance, but they resent their dependence on women" [21].

Men seek ways to overcome their fear. Some men who have sex with men in the United States "report that they get intoxicated [with alcohol or other drugs] precisely because they want to have unsafe sex and are unable to have it when they are sober" [22]. Drinking before visiting brothels in Thailand helps some men overcome the reluctance they would otherwise feel [23]. "There is hope," says Dr Gabriel Kalungi of the Uganda AIDS Commission, referring to the fall in HIV transmission rates, "but alcohol is still a problem. When sober, people are very committed [to protecting themselves] but after drinking at night they seem to think AIDS has disappeared." I.S. Gilada reports that during elections, when sales of alcohol are banned, visits to red-light areas in Mumbai drop by 30 to 40 percent.

In a world where masculine values no longer provide the security that they seemed to provide for their fathers and grandfathers, men's fear is growing. Adriana Gómez, a Chilean feminist, writes that "men are suddenly aware that their marriages are collapsing and leaving them without companionship. They lack emotional ties, they don't have friends and their children don't communicate with them ... They realise that their working life does not always fulfil them and sexuality deprived of affection is little better" [24].

Despair

In the face of HIV, fear may lead to recklessness and despair. In the United States some men who have sex with men take few precautions against infection partly because they expect to contract the virus and partly out of a sense of guilt that they have remained HIV-negative while friends and partners have fallen sick and died; there is almost a sense of relief when a test proves they are HIV-positive [25]. Meshack Ndolo of the Kenyan National AIDS and STD Programme says that "in terms of coping with AIDS, men turn out to be the weaker ones. Most men, when they learn they have HIV, tend to withdraw from circulation, keep away from their friends and, because of that, they tend to die much earlier than women." A similar point is made in the report from Thailand in this book by Phimjai Inthamun of the Community Health Centre in Mae Rim.

A Senegalese doctor suggests that the attitude of women with HIV is "I have to survive, I have to do this or that for my children," while men in the same situation are less motivated. Rose Kolugo-Okwana, who works with TASO (The AIDS Support Organisation) in Uganda, whose services are used by many more women than men, explains that, in general, "Women tend to support each other much more in times of difficulty. They tend to socialise and share out their problems when they go out for other activities like gardening or going for water. Men with HIV lose their status within the community so when they come to know they have the disease, they tend to confine the problem within themselves."

Certainly, in countries – particularly in the West – where most of those who contract HIV are men who have sex with other men, there appear to be more resources for men who fall ill with AIDS than for women. The opposite seems to be true in countries where sex between men and women is the primary means of transmission. One study in Abidjan, Ivory Coast, demonstrates that lower-income women with HIV have access to more resources than men in the same situation. But new approaches are emerging: Uganda has recently seen the formation of POMU (the Positive Men's Union), and New Life Friends Association in northern Thailand supports HIV-positive men in a variety of ways.

"Real men don't get sick"

The need to prove themselves masculine propels men towards risky behaviour; abstinence is seen as unnatural and refusal to use condoms is rationalised in many ways. "It is only really sex when you ejaculate into a woman," says a Zimbabwean man [26]; "'real men' do not get sick," says a Brazilian adolescent [27]. As Mexican sociologists José Aguilar and Luis Botello point out on in this book, condoms represent safety and are therefore inherently unmasculine. Furthermore, they add, "Many young and older men reject [male] condoms because in the middle of sexual conquest they can't put one on without feeling ridiculous."

Many men allege that male condoms reduce sensitivity. This may be true [28], but refusing to wear a condom on such grounds is to suggest that immediate pleasure is more important than the risk of illness and death. Sensitivity can be restored or increased by applying water-based lubricant, where available, to the inside tip of the condom, and prevention programmes across the world have devised means of making condoms both acceptable and erotic.

Even where men are aware that the risk of infection is high and have every opportunity to protect themselves, some are reluctant to do so. As mentioned above, some men who have sex with men in the United States do not use condoms, citing the excitement of 'barebacking'. The impact of their behaviour can be seen in rates of gonorrhoea and syphilis which, after falling in the 1980s and early 1990s, have begun to rise in this group, a statistic which may reflect a rise in rates of HIV [29].

Age, wealth and personality

This picture of men as sexually aggressive, insecure and heedless of the consequences of their actions is painted with a broad brush. Individual attitudes and actions vary widely, and many men consciously or subconsciously reject some or all masculine ideals. Indeed, if the statistics in the previous chapter are accurate, most men's sexual lives place them at little or no risk of contracting and transmitting HIV. Furthermore, other factors such as education, wealth and age can exaggerate or diminish the influence of masculinity on a man's behaviour.

Some men are still unaware of the existence of AIDS: in Bangladesh in 1997, fewer than three adults in 10 had heard of the disease. Knowledge of HIV might be irrelevant if men practised abstinence or used condoms in order to prevent other sexually transmitted infections (STIs) or pregnancy. However, many men consider pregnancy and contraception a problem only for women, while STIs have often been seen as an acceptable risk. Such attitudes, combined with the fact that knowledge of sexual matters is often associated with age and education, mean that the young in particular are at greater risk of contracting infections. WHO estimates that one in every two cases of sexually transmitted disease is in a man or woman under the age of 25, and one in three are in people under the age of 20 [30].

Age may affect a man's risk in different ways. For some, increasing age brings less desire for sex, while for others it brings greater wealth and confidence, and thus more opportunity for intercourse. Wealth is associated with high rates of HIV infection among men in many African societies, although elsewhere wealthy men appear more likely to protect themselves.

Poverty may have both protective and risk-inducing aspects. In some societies poor men tend to have intercourse with fewer women [31]; however, when the opportunity for sex arises, poor men may reject condoms in the belief that the present reward of pleasure or relief is greater than the risk of future illness. And in many countries, homeless or impoverished boys and young men who sell sex in order to survive are unlikely to be able to protect themselves from HIV and other diseases.

Perhaps the biggest influence on men's behaviour is individual personality. Insecurity may place some at risk by the drive to 'prove' themselves through frequent sexual encounters, or insecurity may protect those men who lack the confidence to approach potential sexual partners. Over-confident men who believe no harm can come to them may be less likely to use condoms than men who are careful and cautious in their lives.

Love and lineage

It is paradoxical that in the eyes of many, men's strength dissolves into weakness when they are confronted with their own sexual drive. Certainly, whether or not they are aware of it, masculinity and sex are intertwined throughout many men's lives. As the United Nations Development Programme points out, "Young, single men view sex as a rite of passage and a means of self-exploration, establishing masculinity and building self-esteem ... for some older men, sex is an expression of love and the means of sustaining their lineage; for others it is a means of expressing their virility" [32].

The men in the core groups described in the previous chapter are those who are most likely to adhere to the standards of masculinity described here. Most are probably unaware of the effect of their actions on themselves and their partners. A few, however, who "lie to their partners about their sexual history and even their HIV status, sexually exploit those with less power and use sex as a form of violence" might be described as "irresponsible, selfish and even cruel" [33].

Whether it is the few who act irresponsibly or the many who act unwittingly, all men are threatened by notions of masculinity that place them at risk. Furthermore, contributions to this book from Russia, Brazil, Malawi and elsewhere indicate how HIV and masculinity interact in ways other than sexual behaviour. Yet men are not the only victims; as the following chapter shows, masculinity often has an even greater impact on women.

WOMEN MADE VULNERABLE

Recent years have seen significant improvements in the status of women in many parts of the world. Nonetheless, in comparison with men most women are disadvantaged: women own much less than half the world's property, earn much less than half of global income and generally work considerably longer hours than men.

Many women are not only poorer, but their lives – particularly their sexual lives – are dominated by men. The inability to decide when, how and with whom to have intercourse leaves women vulnerable to a range of serious consequences, including early death from untreated complications in pregnancy or from AIDS and other sexually transmitted infections. Prevention programmes targeted at women have enabled some to protect themselves from the disease, but millions of others will be able to do so only when their male partners are also convinced of the need.

Lifelong depedency

Around the world, perhaps the majority of women spend their lives dependent on men for their survival – first their fathers and brothers, later their husbands, finally their sons or sons-in-law. Dependence on men can affect every aspect of a woman's life, from a childhood in which she receives less food, care and education than her brothers to an adulthood in which she can neither choose her own husband nor the number of children she will bear. Sometimes her dependency is encoded in law, as in those countries where she is denied the right to vote or to inherit or own property. At its most extreme, discrimination against women leads to the abortion of female foetuses and the abandonment of female babies, left to orphanages or even to die.

A young woman may be expected to remain a virgin until she marries the man her father chooses for her, or she may be expected to prove her fertility by becoming pregnant before marriage. Once married, she must remain faithful to her husband, have intercourse with him whenever he wishes and without condoms if he insists; she may have to accept his infidelities and risk violence if she objects. In parts of Africa she is expected to use agents to tighten her vagina or be extremely fastidious in her personal hygiene [1]. In parts of Asia she cannot express pleasure in the sexual act [2].

While the situation is perhaps most extreme in the developing world, many women in industrialised countries, particularly those with relatively low incomes, are similarly affected. For others the pressures may be different. There may be widespread expectations, for example, that a woman's body shape should conform to a specific norm or that women should both work and maintain a household. But whatever the pressures, most are still ultimately driven by men.

Money for new shoes and clothes

Poverty underlies most women's dependence on men and impels them into sexual situations that they might otherwise avoid. In much of sub-Saharan Africa poverty can push women into a range of sexual relationships both before and after marriage, and in many parts of Asia it forces women into unsuitable marriages.

In much of Africa wealth allows men to have many sexual partners, while poverty can force women into the same situation. This attitude is so entrenched that many women and men see no purpose in sexual relationships if financial or other support is not involved. A 20-year-old woman from Ghana says: "After all, what are relationships about then? Men are supposed to provide money and other things. If you don't have money, why do you take a girlfriend in the first place?" A commentator from the same country adds, "No self-respecting woman would enter into a premarital sexual relationship without the potential for material recompense" [3]. In Nigeria sexual networking is also economic networking because it provides women with additional financial security [4], while East African schoolgirls frequently have sex with older men for economic gain. "I needed money to buy new shoes and new clothes," says one 17-year-old from Tanzania, recalling the loss of her virginity at the age of 15.

While many married women remain faithful to their husbands, wives in poorer countries such as Uganda may have several sexual partners in exchange for shelter, food or other means of survival [5]. Women in polygamous unions or young women married to much older men appear more likely to have sex with others because of sexual or emotional needs unmet by their husbands [6]. Such attitudes appear more tolerated in sub-Saharan Africa, where husbands and society may turn a blind eye, and less common in Asia and the Muslim world, where poverty may tie a woman's bonds more closely to her husband.

The lion of the house

Women's submission is often guaranteed by threat of violence. In Uganda 49 percent of sexually active primary schoolgirls report being forced into sexual intercourse [7], while in South Africa 40 to 60 percent of women report regular physical abuse [8]. Young women in India may be beaten and killed by their husband and husband's family if the dowry they bring is considered insufficient, while in Jordan (and elsewhere) women who have been raped are held

Men, Women and Power

It is difficult to make comparisons of men's and women's lives that reflect the reality faced by each individual. In the last 20 years women have become heads of government and of state, and (particularly in industrialised countries) the economic and social gap between women and men is narrowing. Wealth, education, ethnicity and culture play a greater role than gender in the lives of many women, and increasing numbers across the world are free to choose a career, to decide whether, when and whom to marry and to decide whether to divorce.

Thus women with independent income, no matter how meagre, have greater autonomy than women who depend on their husbands for food and shelter, while women whose personalities are stronger than their husbands' have greater control over their lives than women who live in fear. And a woman's relations with some men, such as her sons and younger brothers, may be very different from her relations with her husband, father or elder brothers.

Nor are men's lives always better than women's. As the previous chapter indicated, masculinity can be a burden to men. Men's lifespan is, on average, seven years shorter than women's. Men are more likely to be imprisoned and to die violently and, in the industrialised world, men may face considerably more difficulties than women in education and self-development [15]. There are also areas where comparison between the sexes is difficult, if not impossible. The ability to bear and suckle children, for example, is seen by some as a privilege from which men are excluded, while others consider it a burden that only women have to endure.

"Attributes that are associated with masculinity are not always associated with men. Women, too, can possess some of these attributes," says British commentator Andrea Cornwall. "Not all men, then, have power; and not all of those who have power are men" [16]. Her compatriot Sarah White agrees that concepts of masculinity and femininity cause problems for men as well as for women, but adds that although men may suffer, "they clearly benefit from gender inequality" [17]. ■

in prison for several years in 'protective custody' to prevent their families killing them to expunge the 'dishonour' [9].

Many women who observe domestic violence from a young age excuse it. One Mexican woman said a husband has the right to hit his wife if "the food isn't ready or because he comes home from work and the fire isn't ready" [10]. In Egypt 69 percent of women in one survey said a husband could legitimately beat his wife if she talked back or refused sexual intercourse [11]. Girls from low-income families in Recife, Brazil, dislike violence, but "being bossed around by one's boyfriend is seen by some as proof of love and a sign that their partner is fulfilling his masculine role ... It inspires trust, giving them the sensation that there is a man who will care for them" [12].

Ultimately, therefore, in many relationships men decide and women obey. "I am the lion of the house and [my wife] does not have the right to say no," says one Kenyan man [13]. Poverty and lack of education tend to make women more vulnerable, but others are also at risk. When a middle-class Jamaican woman asked her husband to use a condom, she was told he could find many women who would not make such a request. "I didn't challenge him," she said, "because I don't want to lose him" [14]. It is that fear which places millions of women at risk of contracting HIV.

Pain, love and fear

Young women in particular can be pressured into sex, with consequences that range from emotional hardship to unwanted pregnancies and the devastation of lifelong infection with HIV and probable early death.

Patterns of sexual behaviour differ from culture to culture. If poverty forces many young African women into sexual activity with older men, in Latin America young women are more likely to be pressured into sex by men of a similar age, with unwelcome emotional consequences. One Brazilian survey of first sexual experience found that "pain, love and fear were reported by more than 70 percent of female teens, while pleasure was the overwhelming feeling among male teens" [18]. Throughout the region, "guilty feelings, anxiety over risking a pregnancy and fears of the social consequences of losing one's virginity are some of the feelings at the root of the uneasiness felt by female teens" [19].

Young women's emotional involvement with their partners often prevents them from discussing sex or using condoms. A Brazilian commentator writes that because "the condom creates a sense of strangeness, it symbolises an accusation. Young women say, 'I don't use condoms because I know him'" [20]. Young Thai women tell researchers that "fear of a boy's anger, fear of being looked down on, fear of being perceived that she has had sex before, fear of losing the relationship and fear of being gossiped about prevent girls from communicating about HIV/AIDS, sex and prevention options" [21].

The impact of early intercourse on young women can last a lifetime. Adolescent childbirth has declined in many countries in Asia and the Arab world in recent years, while 30 percent of women in Latin America and over 50 percent in sub-Saharan Africa have their first child before they are 20 [22]. Of even greater consequence, however, is the level of HIV infection, with half of women with the virus contracting it before they reach the age of 25.

Taboos and ignorance

Vulnerability to HIV persists as long as women are sexually active, and is often exacerbated by cultural taboos that encourage or insist that women are ignorant about sexual matters. Married life offers little protection – 20 percent of women with HIV in one study in Kigali, Rwanda, only ever had one partner, while 45 percent of women with the virus contracted it from their husbands [23].

Women of all ages are less likely than men to know that

Sex Work

Women sex workers have been blamed for the spread of HIV, but – as is frequently pointed out – sex work exists only because of the demand from men.

Some women choose sex work to establish economic freedom. Others are forced into it by men who rape them, by parents who sell them to brothel-keepers, or by the loss of their virginity to men who fail to keep their promise to marry them. In other words, inability to earn an independent living, coupled with men's attitudes that women must be 'pure', forces many women into prostitution.

Condom use is becoming more common among sex workers, although many are still unable to persuade clients to use them and others are persuaded to accept extra money for not using them. Sex workers who use condoms with their clients may still be at risk if they are unwilling to use them with their long-term partners. ■

the disease exists, how it is transmitted and how to prevent transmission [24]. "The common belief [is] that to inform girls about sex is to encourage sexual activity," note Brazilian researchers [25], while a similar attitude prevails in northern Thailand [26]. Even where women have knowledge, it may be undermined by men. A 1988 report in *Paris Match* that condoms did not provide complete protection against HIV was read by middle-class men in Zaire who used the 'authority' from a European source as a reason to refuse to protect themselves and their partners [27].

The incidence of sex between men can also place women at risk. Taboos preventing recognition, discussion or acceptance of the practice keep many wives ignorant of their husband's activities. And failure to address the risk of HIV transmission through anal intercourse, with men or women, means that many men are unaware that they should protect themselves and their partners this way.

"That's life"

Women may contract HIV outside or before marriage. In one Thai study up to 20 percent of women, but not their husbands, were shown to be HIV-positive [28]. The way such situations are dealt with depends largely on the attitudes of the individual partners. But it is usually the husband who brings the infection into the family. Even when this is the case, the woman may find herself accused of responsibility for the transmission of the virus [29]. As a result, she may be ejected from her home by the husband or, after his death, by his family.

Rowlands Lenya, director of The Association of People living With AIDS in Kenya (TAPWAK), comments: "We have seen a lot of violence shown to women by men when women test first at ante-natal clinics even if the man is actually responsible for the virus. Where men test HIV-positive first, it becomes easy for the ladies to accept. We tend to think it could be because of the economic situation that sometimes forces women to do this, but I think women in general can cope with difficult situations. When they test HIV-positive they tend to accept faster than the man."

Annelise de Salazar of the Guatemalan Association for the Prevention and Control of AIDS (AGPCS) offers a different opinion: "I don't know if women accept the diagnosis [of HIV/AIDS] more easily. They've lived through a social context where women are always told that they have to take the burden of things. If a woman is beaten, that's life. If a woman is abused, that's part of life. If your husband infects you, that's life – you have to learn to deal with it."

The impact of HIV on women extends beyond their vulnerability to the virus. Women who are HIV-positive may transmit the virus to their new-born children, although zidovudine (formerly known as AZT) reduces the risk to about 1 in 10 births. In the last few years thousands of pregnant women in several developing countries have been offered zidovudine to prevent mother-child transmission. The common practice of withdrawing the drug after the birth and offering the mother no further treatment has been criticised for saving children while probably shortening the lives of their mothers.

Women also tend to take on the responsibility of caring for those who fall sick. This is a time-consuming and labour-intensive task. If they are themselves HIV-positive, the additional work may lead to a deterioration in their own health.

"Within your house, within your bedroom"

Where men appear to be the masters of the house, women may have greater freedom than their husbands suspect. Birth control is one area where men can be unaware of decisions their wives have taken, but HIV prevention, which depends on the man's consent, is more difficult to introduce.

Married women may have some power in sexual relations, but "this must be used subtly, discreetly and indirectly" [30]. A Kenyan woman says: "If you are lucky, you can control your husband, but you control him within your house, within your bedroom" [31]. Many HIV prevention programmes directed at women focus on techniques whereby women whose husbands are impervious to reason can nonetheless achieve their aims through an indirect approach. In the words of a Ghanaian speaker, "He will not accept [the use of condoms] when you are about to do the thing. You wait for the right time when both of you are discussing something else and then you bring it in" [32].

While many observers see women's vulnerability to HIV in terms of male power and female impotence, an alternative analysis is possible. British psychologist Lorraine Sher suggests that women are less likely to leave their partner if he becomes HIV-positive than the other way round; this is commitment, rather than lack of power. Women are less likely to withhold knowledge of their HIV status from their male partner, while HIV-positive men are more likely to keep their female partners in ignorance; this is honesty, not lack of power. And women are more likely to be exposed to unprotected sex from an HIV-positive male partner than the other way round; this is male disregard, not a lack of power [33].

From this perspective it may be that women suffer more because they are able to tolerate more; women, not men, may be the stronger sex. The challenge of the future is to create societies where women's strength achieves its full potential without relegating men to insignificance.

Out of crisis, opportunity

Not every woman is at risk from men's behaviour, and those women who are at risk do not need the example of HIV/AIDS to be told that their lives are to a greater or lesser extent controlled by men. Support groups, whether the informal gathering of women around a well or networks of formally constituted women's organisations, existed long before the epidemic and have analysed the discrepancies between the sexes to much greater depth than is possible in these few pages. Furthermore, many women-orientated groups, such as the Society for Women and AIDS in Africa, have emerged to respond to the threat and consequences of AIDS.

Nevertheless, it is unlikely that women acting alone will bring about a significant change in men's behaviour. The number of women with HIV will continue to rise and may eventually overtake that of men. Increasing numbers will be able to protect themselves from the virus, but without extensive changes in the behaviour of men they probably will remain a minority. The following chapter examines whether millions of men across the social and geographical spectrum can be persuaded to see abstinence, fidelity and the use of condoms as desirable and viable alternatives.

Changing Men's Behaviour

It is clear from the preceding chapters and many of the following reports that men are much more likely to take risks than responsibility in their sexual behaviour. This is not a new phenomenon: centuries of sexually transmitted infections, not to mention the experience of hundreds of millions of men and women the world over, confirm this analysis. But the arrival of HIV/AIDS makes it even more urgent that we confront it.

In the absence of an affordable cure or vaccine, changing men's sexual behaviour is essential to containing the epidemic. The question is how best to achieve that change – a question to which there are no easy answers. Furthermore, since we cannot be certain which men are at risk, we have to address all men.

This chapter gives a brief overview of three approaches to HIV prevention, described here as the 'informative', 'supportive' and 'social'. Experience suggests that the first, directed at men and women and relying solely on information or fear, has little impact, while the second, based on men's images of themselves, has led to some behaviour change. The third approach, which depends on deep-rooted social change, may be the one most likely to overcome the epidemic. It is also the hardest to achieve.

"Use a condom"

In the early days of the epidemic, when it was recognised that AIDS was caused by a sexually transmitted virus, the message in posters and leaflets around the world was simple: abstain from sex, be faithful to your partner or use a condom. Despite widespread publicity in many countries, however, the numbers of those who contract HIV continue to rise.

This is not surprising. Most behaviour that leads to ill-health – such as the sexual transmission of infections, tobacco smoking or poor diet – is at least partly determined by factors that lie outside our conscious control. An informative approach – simply providing information on protection against ill-health – is often insufficient to change behaviour. Tobacco smoking is both a physical and psychological addiction; in some communities poor diet stems from lack of access to the appropriate foods; and, as has been seen, sexual behaviour is determined by a range of factors, including entrenched attitudes and beliefs.

The informative approach has often been supported by messages or images designed to create fear, such as the figure of Death in the first public service announcements on Australian television, the skull that was WHO's first AIDS symbol, and the coffins and emaciated bodies on early leaflets in many countries. While fear may have some impact on behaviour, the general reaction to such images is frequently, "It won't happen to me." Furthermore, associating HIV-positive people with images of death and illness has provoked negative and hostile reactions from the public and led to denial of the possibility of contracting the virus by many of those at risk.

Masculinity and sexual desire

Non-governmental organisations (NGOs) working with groups most at risk, such as men who have sex with men, quickly realised that providing information was not enough and that encouraging fear was counter-productive. Men need support to change their behaviour and the most effective way of doing this is to associate self-protection with attitudes they already hold. Since abstinence and mutual fidelity are not widely admired by men who have sex with men, publicity usually associates condoms with masculinity and sexual

Sexual Options

No programme is likely to succeed if it seeks to impose a specific form of behaviour on its participants or if it reinforces negative masculine traits. Fidelity to one's partner, for example, female or male [5], is a genuine option, but one that relies on open discussion of sexual matters between partners. Fidelity is already achieved probably by the majority of men and could be achieved by many at risk. A study in Mwanza, Tanzania, for example, found that the proportion of men (mainly those older than 25) reporting casual sex partners almost halved over two years, whereas condom use hardly changed [6].

Fidelity gives protection against HIV only if both partners are faithful. In some societies women partners are more likely to be faithful than in others, and in every society male partners are less likely to be faithful than female partners. Achieving mutual fidelity often depends on an ability to discuss sexual matters with one's partner – a discussion which tradition and ignorance may make difficult or near impossible.

Condoms can be an option where fidelity is not, and the appeal to use condoms can be allied with responsibility to a man's present or future family. This can take extreme forms. "I always warn my husband, 'Look, if you are going to one of your parties, remember to carry condoms,'" says one Nigerian woman. "'You know, if you die, I don't eat good. The children will suffer'" [7].

For many men, however, as discussed earlier, a key element of sex is loss of control, an element destroyed by the need to 'interrupt' intercourse to put on a condom. As Vera Paiva, a Brazilian sex educator, explains, "To wear a condom, to be rational, to control sexual drives or take a woman partner's needs into consideration, is to betray maleness" [8]. Some argue that this is a false dichotomy and that condoms do not necessarily symbolise control. An alternative solution is non-penetrative intercourse, which has been promoted with some success, particularly among men in the industrialised world who have sex with men.

Another approach which recognises men's sexual nature is to 'rehabilitate' masturbation. In many countries masturbation is accepted as an appropriate way for young men to release sexual tension; in others, such as Tanzania, it is often seen as a sign of mental weakness, leading many young men to insist on intercourse instead. Yet more openness and acceptance of masturbation as a male activity, as is occurring in Uganda (see following section), almost certainly has some role to play in slowing HIV transmission.

All these approaches – fidelity, condom use, non-penetrative sex, masturbation and abstinence for those not in relationships – are attempts to distinguish between masculinity and sexual prowess. The suggestion is that a man can control and need not be controlled by his sexual appetite. The ultimate goal of HIV prevention and reproductive health may be to divorce the two concepts so that the definition of 'a man' makes no reference to his sexuality. This, it must be acknowledged, is a goal unlikely to be achieved in the near term. ■

desire. This strategy has worked to a certain extent, but not among all men who have sex with men, and not at all times. Infection rates are static, rather than falling, in this group in Australia, the UK and some other countries, and condom use appears to be falling among some US men with many male sexual partners.

The supportive approach relies on publicity and on labour-intensive, lengthy and often costly activities such as individual or group counselling and workshops. In Central America these include 'holistic workshops' for men who have sex with men, which discuss not only HIV transmission but self-confidence, intimacy and alcoholism, leading to greater self-esteem and less willingness to indulge in unsafe sexual behaviour [1]. In a programme in Haiti for men who have sex with women, the Group in Struggle Against AIDS (GLAS) has used 'transactional analysis'. "At first ... the men tended to be concerned only with their own welfare. They often had dominating attitudes towards women," says Glass Aubry, the organisation's director. "Gradually, they began to appreciate that they could get something for themselves by behaving in ways that benefited women" [2].

Women, including sex workers in Africa and housewives in Latin America, have also been the targets of the supportive approach, through discussion groups and one-to-one counselling. The underlying assumption has often been that women can persuade their male partners to use condoms. Some groups of sex workers have agreed not to accept clients without protection and some women have persuaded their partners to use condoms with them or with casual partners. Too often, however, women find that they cannot persuade men; by insisting on condoms, sex workers frequently lose clients, and wives and long-term partners often face violence and rape.

Awareness of this problem has led several programmes to attempt to reach both men and women. Organisations such as the Indian Health Organisation (IHO) arrange counselling for married couples, inviting men to accompany their wives to pre-natal clinics. However, as Dr I.S. Gilada, director of the IHO, admits, no more than 10 to 15 percent of husbands turn up. Similar problems occur in Venezuela, where Nury Pernía of AMBAR (Women's Welfare and Reciprocal Assistance Association) says that for every 20 women at HIV prevention workshops, about 10 male partners will come too. But she adds: "If we succeed in sensitising 10, it's a success."

The Karachi Reproductive Health Project, working in a slum area of Pakistan's largest city, initially ran workshops for men on sexual issues which convinced them that their wives would also benefit from such discussions [3], while in at least one district of Mumbai community elders convinced families to let girls attend sex education sessions [4]. At first sight such a stance may seem to reinforce men's control over women's sexuality, but in the long run it may achieve more fundamental change – if not in the men themselves, then in their sons and daughters.

The consumer culture

By the late 1980s the international donor community had come to recognise the importance of the supportive approach, both through non-governmental initiatives across the world and through social marketing, which uses commercial techniques to promote the sale and use of male condoms. This includes on the one hand a subsidised price and effective distribution, so that condoms are easily accessible to the majority of a population, and on the other hand marketing techniques that associate them with masculinity, such as images of a panther.

Social marketing has achieved sales of tens of millions of male condoms in countries which recorded hardly any condom use a decade ago. A five-fold increase was achieved in Ethiopia (to 21 million sold annually) and a nine-fold increase in Brazil (to 27 million) [9]. Since it is reasonable to assume that people do not pay for a product they do not intend to use, this suggests substantial levels of behaviour change. Social marketing has begun to promote the female condom in Zimbabwe, Brazil and elsewhere.

The technique attracts some critics. Although the condoms have names that promote safety and responsibility, such as 'Trust' and 'Prudence', the overall goal is not to change social attitudes and norms. Behaviour change is promoted without involving men and women in a dialogue that discusses why change is needed and which changes are most appropriate. Furthermore, since marketing research determines condom names and advertising messages, these may reinforce masculine behaviours rather than inviting them to change.

Nevertheless, social marketing reflects the growing trend for consumerism to replace the community as the primary influence on people's lives. Over the last 15 years hundreds of millions of men have been persuaded to drink Coca-Cola, eat McDonald's hamburgers and buy Nike athletic shoes. Commercial companies are successful because they can afford to spend considerable money on research into the most subtle details that influence men's behaviour. Between 1987 and 1997, for example, 70 percent of men in the United States between 25 and 45 years old bought at least one pair of Dockers trousers, persuaded, at least in part, by television advertisements that

With or Without Women?

Men do not live in a vacuum, and since most men are sexually active with women, new definitions of masculinity or adoption of safer sex cannot be achieved without women's participation. However, some men – particularly those who are unpartnered – prefer to discuss sexual issues independently from women. In response to this need, all-male reproductive health clinics have been established in countries from Colombia [11] to Kenya [12]. The experience of a family planning clinic in the United Kingdom, which developed separate facilities for young men and women after considerable tension resulted from both sexes sharing the same space, underlines the importance of adapting education programmes to the needs of those sharing them [13].

Programmes directed at men who have sex with men vary, and approaches that work in one country, or even one community, may not work in another. Appeals to protecting oneself and others on the basis of a gay★ identity, as in the industrialised world or among the middle class of the large cities of Brazil or Argentina, have little impact in communities where the concept of a gay identity is unknown or even denied. In Dhaka, Bangladesh, for example, the Bandhu Social Welfare Society explicitly rejected this approach when working with lower-income men, many of whom are married, who have sex with other men.

Whatever the approach, HIV prevention cannot be divorced from other aspects of reproductive health, such as pregnancy and sexually transmitted infections. "When reproductive health decisions are taken jointly by both partners, these decisions are more likely to be implemented," say specialists Isaiah Ndong and William Finger [14]. The statement is true whether the partners' commitment lasts for life or 10 minutes. As a family planning study from Johns Hopkins University in Baltimore, US, concludes: (i) learn what men want and need (ii) present men as caring partners, not adversaries (iii) encourage men to talk to their partners and make joint decisions (iv) publicise and promote service sites for men (v) work with opinion leaders (vi) work with young men and (vii) continue to learn [15]. ■

★   That is, men who have sex with men. See the report from Kenya below for a fuller definition of 'gay'.

responded to their self-esteem and recognised the ways in which they process information and the fact that many lack self-confidence [10]. Unfortunately, the financial and creative resources available for sexual health initiatives are far fewer than those available to the commercial sector.

The social approach

Whatever the benefits and problems associated with social marketing, even its backers acknowledge that it is not enough on its own. "It is clear that we have increased use, that we have met a demand that emerged with AIDS," says Guy Stallworthy, director of technical services for Population Services International, a US-based non-profit organisation that coordinates many of the world's largest social marketing campaigns. "But is there a plateau effect taking place? Are we able to persuade more people to use condoms? To increase sales at this point, we have to change societal norms" [16].

Changing societal norms (the social approach) means recognising the context of men's lives, addressing their fears and desires and encouraging responsibility, communication with partners and respect for others and oneself. This is a time-consuming, uncertain process that relates not only to HIV/AIDS but to the many broader issues surrounding gender relations that have come to the fore in recent years, especially since the adoption of the international Convention on the Elimination of All Forms of Discrimination Against Women (CEDAW) in 1979. The discussion here, however, is restricted to aspects which affect masculinity and HIV.

What sort of norms can society move towards? Can masculinity be more strongly associated with responsibility and masculine values become a basis for protecting oneself, one's partner(s) and one's family? As Patricia Burke of the Jamaican National AIDS Committee says, "If men can be encouraged to value sexual responsibility and restraint rather than excess, we will have gone a long way toward reducing the risk" [17]. Can masculinity and sexual prowess be divorced, so that a man's respect for himself and other men does not depend on sexual activity?

Terms of debate

Effective and long-lasting change within any society can come only from full and informed debate. Such a debate on masculine values depends on a number of principles, the first of which is that change cannot be imposed from outside, whether by the international community on national AIDS activities, or by national AIDS programmes or political or religious leaders on individual men. Institutions and individuals from outside a society, including those who work on HIV, development, human rights, gay issues or religion, can provide the resources which allow the debate to take place, but they cannot impose resolutions or prejudge outcomes.

As a second principle, the debate must include individuals who may be marginalised by society; those most affected by HIV, directly or indirectly, are often those most marginalised by society: women, drug injectors, men who have sex with men, men and women who have contracted the virus. Continuing to marginalise rather than assist those at risk may satisfy a current moral stance, but by allowing the epidemic to spread, it contravenes the deeper moral imperative of preserving life. Attempting to impose solutions on people who cannot accept them is likely to drive the epidemic underground.

Thirdly, the discussion over what it means 'to be a man' must take place in public and in private, in formal settings and informal networks. This means between husbands and wives, between individual men, in their homes or in groups facilitated by a range of NGOs. The debate must also take place within institutions, such as NGOs, commerce, the media, the church, mosque and temple, as well as the formal settings of national and state parliaments and other political assemblies.

Fourthly, the debate cannot exclude topics on grounds of 'morals' or 'taste'. Inability to talk about sex has led to widespread ignorance, false perceptions and impossible ideals. The consequences of ignorance are severe. Lack of knowledge of sexually transmitted infections prevents millions of women and men from seeking treatment, leading to serious health risks for themselves, their partners and their children. But many authorities appear unable to support open and effective HIV prevention programmes. Government-sponsored billboards in Bangladesh, for example, picture deserted villages and advise people to 'avoid AIDS', without indicating how the disease is transmitted or how to prevent transmission.

Men, therefore, need the opportunity to discuss what it means 'to be a man', why they use their penis, mouth or anus in certain ways, what they expect from their sexual partners, what they believe they owe their partners, what gives them pleasure or brings them pain. Women must have the same freedom. The language may vary, depending on the setting – the bedroom, the community workshop, the magazine or newspaper or the national assembly – but the subject cannot be censored if there is to be genuine scope for change.

Finally, the greatest challenge in HIV prevention is for those men who hold the reins of power in society – as parliamentarians, religious leaders, newspaper editors and broadcast producers, as fathers and husbands – to recognise that this is the moment to enable others to determine their own behaviour and fate. In doing so, many will discover that they too have been burdened by expectations that have restricted their ability to determine their own lives. This does not mean that men with power should be silent. As Meschack Ndolo of the Kenyan National AIDS and STD Control Programme says, "We need to get the participation of the community stakeholders, most of whom are men, the

No to Marginalisation

There is a strong correlation between social support and safer sex. Lonely, isolated gay men in Norway appear less likely to use condoms than those who live in a supportive environment; perceptions that their parents care for them are more likely to encourage US teenagers to protect themselves than warnings about health risks [18].

The World Bank calls on governments to support all risk-reducing preventive interventions, from lowering the price of condoms to teaching drug users to sterilise injecting equipment [19]. The Brazilian government supports prevention programmes for men who have sex with men, and authorities from Nepal and Vietnam to the United Kingdom either actively support or allow needle exchange programmes.

In many communities those who have contracted HIV are subject to stigmatisation and rejection, even where the virus is widespread [20], but as Satya Sivaraman's report from Thailand points out, men and women living with HIV/AIDS can play a positive role in preventing further dissemination of the disease. People who are HIV-positive have first-hand knowledge of how and why people contract the virus and its impact on their lives. As UNAIDS says, "Community-level action – much of it initiated by persons infected or affected by HIV – has always played a major role in the global response to AIDS" [21]. ∎

custodians of traditions." But it does mean they should recognise that those who are most affected by the epidemic are those who understand best how to prevent its transmission.

The present challenge

Debates over the role of men in HIV prevention and how to enable men to change their behaviour have already begun in many countries, in private, in NGOs and academia, occasionally in the media and elsewhere. In only a few countries such as Uganda, however, is the attempt to discuss the sexual behaviour and responsibilities of men and women throughout society seen as a priority for society as a whole.

More often the debate is ignored, and – particularly when women assume leadership roles in HIV prevention – disparaged. Eka Esu-Williams, president of the Society of Women and AIDS in Africa, points out that "typical responses [from community leaders, most of whom are men] include the notion that women working on HIV/AIDS are feminists or want to be liberated ... Policy-makers are not often enthusiastic about supporting women's groups fighting ... HIV/AIDS because they might address issues which are not thought to be appropriate or would press for the rights of women. Women [working in HIV prevention] can feel insecure and unsafe, believing that addressing HIV/AIDS would stigmatise them and would make people think they are infected." In short, millions of men and women must die because the men who lead our communities are afraid of change, and of yielding or sharing power.

So the debate is difficult. It goes to the heart of the identity of individuals and societies. In many countries the temptation is to refuse to debate, to insist that the solution to HIV prevention can be found within already existing structures and values. Yet the truth is that existing structures and values have allowed the epidemic to spread in country after country, continent after continent, out of control.

No going back

The clock cannot be turned back to a time when there was no HIV. Nor can the world return to some mythical period where all men and women were celibate before marriage and faithful thereafter. The long history of other sexually transmitted infections is proof that no society has ever seen such a golden age.

Ultimately, changes in men's behaviour are likely to result from broader social forces than HIV/AIDS prevention, although increasing awareness of HIV/AIDS is likely to play a significant role in influencing these broader forces. The gradual shift in emphasis in many cultures from the extended family and community to the individual may have contributed to the spread of HIV, but in the long run it may lead to men's willingness to protect themselves and others. As the Humsafar Trust, an NGO in India, writes, citing WHO research, "People make positive choices about their sexual health when they have a strong sense of self and identity and personal/family responsibility" [22].

Achieving this, however, will be a complex task. As the following chapters indicate, individual men's lives differ considerably across the globe. They range from men who consider it their right to abuse their wives both physically and sexually to men who are physically and sexually abused by other men; from men who struggle to reconcile their faith with their sexual desires to men who struggle to survive with HIV; from young men whose lives are driven by their next drug injection to young men with no cares, plenty of money and plenty of women on whom to spend that money. Men who place themselves and others at risk present a challenge, for at the same time they must be confronted with the impact of their behaviour and given the considerable support they need to help them to change.

Eleven countries are represented in the following chapters. In each a specific situation is portrayed. This does not mean that the situation described is the greatest problem that country faces from the epidemic; what it does mean is that many of these countries represent problems that are widespread elsewhere. Domestic violence is by no means restricted to Mexico; the conditions in Brazilian prisons are found across the world; Kenya is not the only country in Africa or elsewhere where the authorities refuse to acknowledge the existence of men who have sex with men; armed forces across the world face the same problems as those in Malawi; the experience of reaching large groups of men in Bangladesh can be used throughout the world.

Although the focus of this book is men, women must remain clearly within the picture. As HIV prevention for women cannot succeed without the active involvement of men, prevention for men is meaningless without the participation of women. It is the hope of the authors of this work that it should help encourage the debate that will lead to greater understanding of the complex relationship between the sexes, and to widespread effective prevention of HIV and other sexually transmitted infections.

PART TWO

WHEN WOMEN SAY NO

INTRODUCTION

In Latin America concepts of masculinity are encapsulated in the word machismo. *At its most extreme, machismo maintains a man's superiority over women, granting him the freedom to do as he pleases within and outside the family home and the authority to restrict the freedom of his wife and daughters. Machismo ensures that only the man can experience pleasure during sex; women who do so are considered shameless or arouse suspicion in their husband that they have had experience with other men. Constantly afraid that their wives will fall from grace, Mexican* machos *subscribe to the saying that: "Women are like shotguns: they should be kept loaded [pregnant] and indoors."*

Machismo appears to be strength, but machista *attitudes are often no more than the armour men wear to protect their weaknesses. As one specialist in gender relations writes, "Most men feel ... impotent. Even though they know that the definition of masculinity is being in power, being 'the captain of my fate and master of my soul', they feel trapped in old, suffocating roles, unable to make the changes they want in their lives" [1]. This sense of impotence frequently leads to violence, perpetuating a pattern in which men who were beaten as boys by fathers and who saw their fathers beat their wives react to challenges to their authority in the only way they know.*

Men's aggression towards women is by no means unique to Latin America. The number of women who say that they have experienced domestic violence [2] ranges from 20 percent in China, through 25 percent in Belgium and Norway, over 40 percent in Guatemala, Kenya and Uganda, to 80 percent in Pakistan [3]. In Mexico half of all women can expect to be hit by their long-term partners during their lifetime. At its most extreme, domestic violence leads to death: research indicates that nearly half of all murder victims in Russia in 1995 were women murdered by their male partners, while in the United States "10 women are killed by their batterers every day" [4].

Growing awareness of domestic violence led to adoption of the United Nations Declaration on the Elimination of Violence Against Women in 1993, and some countries, including Mexico, have taken steps to implement laws intended to protect women. However, such laws are simply the first in a series of steps that must be taken to protect women and enable men to overcome the fears and insecurities that lead them to attack their partners.

Rape aside, HIV is transmitted not through violence but through the fear that prevents wives from asking their husbands to desist from extra-marital affairs or to use a condom. In this first of two reports on relations between men and women, Eda Chávez looks at the lives of ordinary Mexicans and the attendant risks of transmitting HIV.

DOMESTIC VIOLENCE AND HIV/AIDS IN MEXICO
by Eda Chávez

Mexico is a vibrant, complex country in the throes of social change. Five hundred years of European heritage have blended with rich native tradition; these elements in turn are increasingly overshadowed by the influence of its powerful neighbour, the United States. Millions of peasants speaking indigenous tongues consider they are treated as second-class citizens compared to the Spanish-speaking majority, and in urban neighbourhoods poverty and great wealth sit side by side. Once persecuted and still denied official status, the Roman Catholic Church commands the religious loyalty of nine tenths of the population, from illiterate farmers to the political elite, while 70 years of one-party rule have finally given way to municipal, state and federal elections won by opposition candidates from both sides of the political spectrum.

Political change may be widespread but social attitudes remain highly conservative. There is strong hostility towards any challenge to the sexual status quo, particularly in areas where the conservative National Action Party (PAN) forms the government. This has hindered HIV/AIDS prevention work in many places. In 1995 the police in Tlaquepaque barred public distribution of condoms. In the same year a hospice for the terminally ill in Guadalajara was closed on the pretext that classes were being given in safer sex. And in 1997 women in Ciudad Juárez were charged with "offences against public morality and good custom" for putting up AIDS posters.

Such attitudes are not new. They are merely the latest manifestation of a deep-rooted machismo that for generations has allowed men to consider women as little more than objects of desire. The majority of women remain resigned and obedient, enjoying little or no say in sexual matters and facing the very real risk of violence from their partners if they attempt to assert their independence and control over their own bodies.

Sex and violence

"I knew Antonio was having affairs with other women but he told me he always used protection with them. That was the only time I dared to ask him to use a condom. I shouldn't have! He hit me several times, even though I was pregnant."

Norma, Mexico City

Although the subject has not been investigated systematically, there is enough evidence from individual studies to suggest that violence forms an integral part of the lives of many Mexican women. Surveys indicate that 53 percent of respondents from urban areas and 42 percent from rural areas have been subject to violence at least once in their lives [5]. In one group of women 75 percent had been subject to physical violence and 45 percent had suffered sexual violence [6]. According to the office of the Attorney General in Mexico City, between October 1990 and April 1994 there were almost 89,000 victims of domestic violence [7].

Violence often starts while the woman is still a child, and is perpetrated by the father or by brothers. "I finished primary school and they didn't let me continue, because I was a girl. I was prohibited from speaking to men. One day a boy asked me the time just as my brothers happened to pass by. They knocked me around like crazy" [8]. Leaving home to escape from violence is not always the solution. "I left with a boy in order to escape from my house where my father and my brothers beat me. But I have suffered so much with my husband because he has also beaten me all my life and abused me" [9].

Researchers from the Pan American Health Organization (PAHO) point out that society encourages women to be dependent and submissive and men to be violent and aggressive. "Not only are boys allowed to be openly aggressive and fight with their fists, but this type of behaviour is expected of them" [10]. Adult men learn to use violence "competitively with their equals and oppressively with their 'inferiors'"; women learn to live with it [11].

Sex often lies at the heart of domestic violence – a man's suspicion that his wife is having sex with another man, or a woman's desire not to have sex when her partner wishes. In both cases the violence stems from the man's fear that he is losing control of 'his' woman. Norma, quoted above, lived with her husband for 11 years from the age of 15; during that time, "he wouldn't even let me walk to the end of the street on my own." Another woman's experience is that, "My feelings didn't matter at all. He took me by force, and if I didn't want to, he hit me, and the next day he didn't leave me alone until I would go with him again" [12]. The man's perspective is evident in the words of Jorge, 39: "Sometimes she doesn't want to, but in the end she gives in. I have to

How Many Women?

The statistics on HIV transmission in Mexico may be unclear, but there is no dispute that married women are at risk of contracting the virus. At the beginning of 1998 the National Council for the Prevention of AIDS (CONASIDA, a government body) estimated that between 159,000 and 212,000 Mexicans (approximately four in every 1,000 adults) were living with HIV.

At least 25,000 women are believed to be HIV-positive, although the number may be much higher. Experts disagree about the profile of the epidemic. In most countries it is usual to assume that the pattern of HIV transmission is similar to that of cases of AIDS. In Mexico, however, analysis is complicated by the fact that in a high proportion of cases (41 percent in 1996) the method of transmission is unknown. Whether these unknown cases are ignored, allocated to sex between men, to sex between men and women, or to drug injection radically alters the picture.

Some researchers believe that the high figure of 'unknowns' masks a considerable amount of transmission between men, since hostility towards men who are penetrated by other men is so high that few admit to the practice. AIDS specialist José Antonio Izazola claims that "the homosexual face of the epidemic is being covered in order to make it respectable in the eyes of Mexican people." His comments reflect the quandary faced by the health authorities, who on the one hand wish to avoid stigmatising AIDS as a 'homosexual disease', but on the other hand face the accusation that the attempt to de-stigmatise the disease is a ploy to justify lack of government action to protect men who have sex with men.

CONASIDA recognises that more men than women have contracted HIV, but points out that the epidemic has several faces in Mexico. In some states, such as Baja California, Jalisco and Sonora, injecting drug users account for up to 15 percent of AIDS cases. Other states, such as Michoacán, Tlaxcala and Hidalgo, have many cases in rural areas closely linked to migration to and from the United States. The epidemic is spreading fastest in rural areas, where it is doubling every six or seven months, compared to every 16 to 18 months in urban areas [17].

The pattern of HIV transmission among women has changed dramatically. Originally most women contracted the virus from transfusions of contaminated blood, but heterosexual transmission is now the leading cause. The women most affected are not sex workers, who are generally aware of the risk and can take steps to protect themselves (transmission rates in this group have remained consistently below one percent for several years), but women who have been faithful to their husbands and are either unaware of the risk or unable to protect themselves. With 1,800 women diagnosed with AIDS in the first eight years of the epidemic, and the same number diagnosed in the subsequent three years, the epidemic among women is more recent but is growing faster than among men. ■

insist and make her, but finally she gives in."

If sex is the cause, alcohol is often the trigger. Much domestic violence occurs when the man is drunk and less open to reason. The experience of Juana, a 32-year-old divorced street trader, is typical: "My husband is alcoholic. He almost always arrived home drunk from work and forced me to have sex with him. He never bothered to ask. Then I learned I had HIV and it was he who gave it to me."

One study of the health problems that result from persistent violence in the home showed that one in three women suffered from emotional distress or other mental disorders and one in 10 from gynaecological problems. While not every emotional state or illness can be blamed on domestic violence, there is clearly a correlation. "I have had a problem with chronic conjunctivitis. I think it's from crying so much. Now I have a lot of headaches." "I have constant muscle pains and rheumatism and headaches. I'm always anxious and upset." "Lately I've had dizziness, headaches, menstrual problems." "I get needle-like headaches, frequent dizziness and my vision gets cloudy. I feel like crying over anything" [13].

Perhaps because it is so widespread, domestic violence is often seen as 'normal'. The victim is blamed, or the situation is ignored because it is considered part of a couple's private life. As PAHO points out, "For centuries, violence against women within the family has been considered 'natural'. Traditionally, married women have been viewed as the 'property' of the husband, who had the right to discipline his wife just as he did his children" [14]. Because a man is theoretically responsible for maintaining order in the home, he is unlikely to be punished for striking his wife or companion. In PAHO's words, "The weakness of the judicial system in condemning the violence of men toward women in private ultimately serves to sanction such violence, creating the image that it can be an acceptable means for controlling women" [15].

Men's analysis of their own violence sometimes expresses awareness that what they do is wrong and sometimes cites the woman's behaviour as justification. Juan Carlos, a 40-year-old former policeman, says that he hit his wife "because the devil took hold of me and she set the children against me." Eduardo Liendro of CORIAC (Collective of Men for Equal Relationships) points out that even those who regret their actions can find it difficult to stop. Liendro claims that men are also victims, although they physically suffer less: "It's difficult for men to feel good when we repress our emotions, when we are causing pain and alienating those we love ... We have sought escape valves, such as sport, alcohol, drugs, violence against other men" [16].

Afraid of their partners, with little hope of support from the community or the law, women often refuse to denounce their husband's violence for fear of further attacks. A study from the Interdisciplinary Women's Studies group at the College of Mexico concludes that the fear, shame and humiliation of ill-treatment force women to continue the relationship even when it becomes more violent. In the words of Imelda, Juan Carlos's wife, "If I tell the police, he will only get more angry and things will get worse when he returns."

Many women stay in relationships because they depend on

their male partners for economic security for themselves and their children. Furthermore, a woman's fear of retaliation against herself, her children and others who support her; her hope that her partner will change, based on the man's own promises; and the potential for shame and blame from priests, police officers, health workers, friends and others all prevent her from leaving her partner or reporting the abuse.

Fear and ignorance

"I remember three women who had contracted HIV from their husbands. What upset them most was the incredible frustration of trying to understand how a man can love and at the same time hold out his hand in welcome and lead to death. They were totally disillusioned by the men who had once stood by their side."

Marisol Martínez, lawyer with COVAC
(Collective to Fight Violence Against Women)

Irrespective of the actual numbers of women who have contracted the virus, machismo and fear of violence clearly have a role to play in HIV transmission in Mexico. Some women have become HIV-positive only because they have been faithful to their partners. Norma, quoted above, recently discovered she had the virus. Her partner, whom she has since left, "was the only person who could have passed the virus to me." Others have known that their partners were unfaithful but have been unable to demand the use of a condom. Eduardo Liendro believes that fear of AIDS has worsened sexual violence within marriage as women try to protect themselves: "When women don't want to have sex with their husband for whatever reason, many men force them to."

Meanwhile, machismo is reinforced by and reinforces ignorance. Sex education in schools, the family and the mass media is minimal. In rural areas, especially, all talk of sex is taboo, except for men claiming sexual conquests. "I resolved all my questions [about sex] partly through practice and partly through older friends or their brothers, because nobody talked about it in my house, far less at the school I went to, which was run by priests," remembers Alberto Andrade, a 38-year-old clerk.

Women are expected to have little or no awareness of sexual issues. Norma was surprised to discover that she had contracted HIV, although she knew her husband had other partners, because "he was always very particular about personal hygiene." In common with many others she believed that cleanliness provided protection against sexually transmitted disease.

Ignorance is considered normal, according to Susan Pick, director of the Mexican Institute of Family Research, leading people to experience anxiety, guilt or fear when they want to inform themselves and resolve their doubts about their sexuality. "As long as society's attitude towards sexuality continues to be that of prohibition, it will continue to be difficult to teach young people and adults to negotiate safer sexual practices with their partner and it will impede a natural and open education of boys and girls towards a mature and responsible sexuality."

Minimising machismo

Changing attitudes as entrenched as machismo in a population of more than 90 million is not an easy task. Steps are being taken at a number of levels to limit the spread of HIV and to reduce the incidence of domestic violence. In late 1997, half a century after a similar law failed to reach the statute books, the government made it illegal for a man to beat or rape his wife.

Passing a law, however, is very different from enforcing it. Marisol Martínez, a lawyer working for COVAC, claims the new legislation is a significant advance in that it subjects husbands who commit sexual violence against their wives to the same penalties (eight to 14 years' imprisonment) as other men convicted of the same crime. However, Martínez adds, in the first four months that the law was in effect, "none of the cases of which I am aware have led to proceedings for domestic violence as specified in the penal code."

Non-governmental organisations (NGOs) have limited resources, but they can work with many individuals on issues of machismo and HIV/AIDS. COVAC provides legal, emotional and psychological support for women who have been subject to domestic, including sexual, violence. CORIAC began workshops on reducing male violence in 1993. According to Eduardo Liendro, "Men come when they are in crisis, recently separated or beginning a second relationship which is not working out, or because they have struck their partner and they were shocked to discover they had reached that point. Others are motivated by their partners, by the implication 'If you don't go, we'll split up'" [18]. Many women also seek CORIAC's assistance, and the collective has established a programme which helps women develop and maintain self-esteem, a necessary first step in asserting themselves or leaving abusive relationships.

CORIAC's strategy is first to point out to the men the risks they face from machista attitudes – the stress that comes from insisting on retaining control and which leads to ill-health and heart attacks – and then to make them aware of when they are under stress and help them to deal with it. "The first thing we give are very concrete tools," explains Liendro, "to recognise the fatal risk and to know what has to be done to retreat and change. If I recognise that I feel bad because of something my partner has said or done, I have to take a step back, get out of the place where this thing that is disturbing me is happening, for an hour or more, without taking a drink, without driving, without reaching for a weapon, without going to another woman ... All this is a basic technique for reducing the tension which can lead to violence. In the first session we also teach men breathing and relaxation exercises for them to do during this hour which allows time to think" [19].

CORIAC is not always successful in changing attitudes. "We are aware," says Liendro, "that while some men believe they have progressed to the point where they have eliminated violence from their lives, their partners do not always see this progress as so evident" [20].

Colectivo Sol works with men who have extramarital affairs with women and men. Juan Jacobo Hernández, the director, points out some of the difficulties in devising campaigns in this field: "Who should the campaign be directed at? The man who has unprotected sex or the wife, so that both can agree to use condoms? By intervening in a relationship you are entering dangerous territory. There are problems here that do not yet have a solution."

Real men don't – or do – use condoms

"Having sex with a condom is like eating mole *[a national dish] with gloves,"*

Marcos, Mexico City

In 1997 CONASIDA launched the third national AIDS prevention campaign, with advertising 'spots' broadcast throughout the country by 92 television stations and 1,173 radio stations, as well as 150,000 posters in well-frequented places such as the capital's metro system. The focus was on encouraging condom use among adolescents of both sexes, although there has been concerted opposition to condoms from the Catholic Church.

For many young men condoms are a barrier to affirming their virility. According to sociologists José Aguilar and Luis Botello, "many young and older men reject condoms because in the middle of sexual conquest they can't put on a rubber without feeling ridiculous." In a series of interviews for this report, of 50 men aged between 15 and 48 in Oaxaca and Mexico City, only 10 percent consistently used condoms. None used condoms with their wives or regular girlfriends, although 15 percent admitted that their partners had asked them to do so.

Men can find many reasons for not using *gomitas, guantes, sombreritos* – 'rubbers'. Some claim, often wrongly, that they are not at risk of contracting a disease. "I don't use a condom because I don't go to bars where there are prostitutes. I only do it with my wife or with girls," says Pedro, a 23-year-old salesman from Oaxaca state. Jorge, a 28-year-old teacher in a rural school, uses condoms only to avoid pregnancy: "I trust myself and my partner." Guillermo, a 39-year-old labourer is also married and unfaithful, "but I always check that they are clean and so I don't always have to use a condom." Others suggest that machos do not fall ill: "The only ones who catch these diseases are the ones who aren't man enough," says Juan, a 55-year-old taxi driver.

Nonetheless, there are signs of change. According to CONASIDA condom use is most common amongst sexually active men aged between 15 and 19, with 44 percent using condoms at least occasionally in their sexual encounters. In general, young men first use condoms within a year of becoming sexually active, in order to prevent transmission of disease. This is a change from the previous generation, who began to use condoms in their mid-twenties, 10 years after their first sexual relationship, in order to prevent pregnancy.

For some middle- and upper-class adolescents, a condom reflects masculinity, although they may buy them for status more than for sex. "For a young man to carry a condom affirms his masculinity and gives him prestige in his social group," assert Aguilar and Botello, a point reaffirmed by 19-year-old Luis, who says: "My friends only carry a condom to claim that they are having sexual relations."

This is nonetheless an important first step, and one which Aguilar and Botello believe should be taken further. Since belonging to a group of 'ideal' (or dominant) men is more important than disease prevention for most young men, they recommend associating condoms with virility and masculinity. They also recommend including gender in the education of children and young adults, as "an opportunity to break the paradigm of the 'ideal (machista) man' and to slowly internalise the 'real man', given that it is in early youth that identity is consolidated and it is the moment to construct new masculinities" [21].

Most radically, Aguilar and Botello propose promoting condoms for masturbation. This would not only "increase the ability to use condoms, but would internalise the values of looking after oneself and knowing one's own body, values currently not permitted to the ideal man."

Signs of change

Although a legal battle has been won in terms of the criminalisation of domestic violence and marital rape, Mexican woman are still far from winning the war of sexual emancipation. But "if there is a positive side to AIDS, it is that it provides proof that the very unequal relationship between men and women in poor countries is a danger for the human race," says Ana Luisa Liguori of the US-based MacArthur Foundation. Indeed, AIDS has opened a window of opportunity for men and women to begin to think and seriously discuss how to break ancient patterns of behaviour which are having such a negative impact on the eve of the 21st century.

Men's attitudes towards women and their belief in machismo may be changing, particularly among the younger generation. Fathering many children, for example, is no longer essential to proving one's manhood, according to Toño, a 27-year-old car mechanic from Mexico City: "Having a lot of kids to prove you're macho is bullshit. These ideas are 40 years old" [22].

Patricia Duarte Sánchez and Gerardo González, co-founders of COVAC, see light at the end of the tunnel. "In addition to providing services and engaging in the legal reform process, feminists have also managed to involve the government and broad sectors of the population in a wider discussion of gender relations. Today, as a result of all these efforts, [awareness of] gender violence is no longer confined to the private sphere. It is a public issue that is debated in academia, in labour unions and political parties, in grassroots organisations, in the urban movement and in professional schools" [23]. The writers point out that many branches of government, from the Ministry of Education to the Ministry of the Interior, from attorney-generals to family welfare programmes, have developed policies which recognise the impact of gender violence and which attempt to remove its causes.

Changing Times?

INTRODUCTION

HIV has spread rapidly in eastern Africa in the last 15 years, and Tanzania has been particularly hard hit. Chrysostom Rweyemamu's report confirms that many of the factors behind the global epidemic are present in the country, including men's dominance, infrequent condom use, early sexual initiation and high rate of partner change. It is possible that the last two are the product of extensive urbanisation and migration in the last 40 years, but the few studies that have examined this issue have given contradictory results.

If it is difficult to measure sexual activity, it is even more difficult to summarise attitudes towards it. Nevertheless, Rweyemamu captures the ambivalence that many Tanzanians feel about their sexual lives and the often wide discrepancy between their ideals and reality. Sometimes the men and women he interviews suggest that intercourse is an activity which both sexes freely enjoy; sometimes it is characterised as a man's right and a woman's duty; at other times, particularly when age and wealth meet youth and poverty, it emerges as a bargaining tool. Tradition, in the form of widow inheritance and avoidance of pregnant women or women who have just given birth, also plays a role.

In many ways, therefore, Tanzania typifies relations between men and women in countries with few resources and illustrates many of the points described in the introduction to this book. The comments of ordinary men and women make it clear how difficult it is to promote condom use, abstinence and fidelity when so many factors drive sexual activity. Nonetheless, there is some indication that the rate of HIV transmission has begun to fall in parts of Tanzania. If the comments of young people here are typical, 10 years from now the picture will be much more optimistic.

SEXUAL BEHAVIOUR IN TANZANIA

by Chrysostom Rweyemamu

According to the Joint United Nations AIDS Programme (UNAIDS), an estimated 940,000 Tanzanians have died from AIDS and 1.4 million – almost one adult in 10 – are living with HIV. Yet although most people are aware of the disease and its modes of transmission, there appears little sense of urgency or fear. Dr KJJ Kashaija of the Tanzania Red Cross believes people have become indifferent to the disease, rationalising high risk behaviour through proverbs such as *okaluga omubibelo noija kugwa omubibelo* ('You came from a woman's thighs and you will die in a woman's thighs'), which suggest that death is inevitable and AIDS is the will of God.

Indeed, for many Tanzanians there are more important problems than HIV/AIDS. "When I wake up in the morning my worry is always whether I will get work for that day to enable me to get something for my family's survival," says Ananias, who sometimes finds work washing clothes and sheets in Muhimbili Medical Centre in the capital, Dar es Salaam. "Whenever I have sex, my worry is more about the chances of getting pregnant than about the risk of contracting AIDS," says 19-year-old Sherida, a hairdresser in Dar es Salaam. "Now my boyfriends have got used to me they no longer use condoms," she adds, apparently unaware that her boyfriends, Raymond and Hassan, have other girlfriends and the chances are that these girlfriends have other sexual partners who do not use condoms.

Second-class citizens

Sherida's admission that she has two boyfriends is a far cry from the traditional behaviour expected of a young Tanzanian woman. Tribal customs and the Christian and Muslim religions all dictate that both men and women should be chaste before marriage and loyal to their spouses thereafter.

Traditionally, however, men have been allowed greater latitude than women. In the past, "female chastity was so highly valued [by the Haya tribe] that unmarried pregnant girls were thrown into Lake Victoria," says 57-year-old Melchior Toroto, who lives near Muleba town. Toroto points out that although boys were also expected to refrain from sex before marriage, they did not suffer such drastic punishment. They also benefited from greater sexual freedom after marriage, since Islam and many tribal customs allowed a husband more than one wife. The practice remains, with one in four women and one in six men in polygynous marriages [1].

Generally, girls and women have been valued less in themselves than as mothers, particularly the mothers of sons. Joyce Christina Kafanabo of the Civil Service Department's Gender Unit in Dar es Salaam points out that even today female babies are often a cause of disappointment to a family. In some regions, if a couple are childless after five years of marriage or their only offspring are girls, the husband is free to seek a son through another woman. The implication is that the woman is at fault, although men, too, may be sterile and it is the man's sperm, not the woman's ovum, that decides the sex of the child.

According to Kafanabo, "Women experience domination and discrimination that last a lifetime." Girls are fed less than their brothers and are allocated household tasks and social roles that men refuse. Typically, Kafanabo says, a woman "works for unequal pay, and has the double burden of work at home and on the job. She has no control over her body and she lives in fear of violence."

Dancing to the tune of her husband

Traditional attitudes between the sexes persist in many parts of Tanzania. "For a woman to be dominated by a man is one of God's plans," says Sheikh Mohammed Abdallah, 56. "That is why no woman is allowed to decide when to have sex."

"I am legally married to my wife and if I have sex with her when she is not ready, that is not rape. A woman is there to serve and dance to the tune of her husband, full stop," insists Ali Kagashe, 47. "A woman has to service a man any time he wants her. That's why God created her – to be submissive to a man, who is always stronger than her. In a nutshell, she belongs to the kitchen," asserts Gadiel Komuka, a peasant in Muleba district.

Men's domination can turn to violence. "My neighbour is openly running around with several women while his wife has been told to keep quiet on the issue," says Gosbert Rubona, a civil servant in Dar es Salaam. "Recently his wife gathered courage and humbly advised him to take care not to contract HIV. The reward for this advice was a severe beating in which her right eye was so badly damaged that it had to be removed."

Even without the threat of violence, few Tanzanian women refuse sex. "For a girl to say 'no' to her lover or boyfriend depends on special circumstances, say when she is on her period or when she is sick," says retired teacher Imelda Kiwelu. "If this is not the case, she can't afford to say 'no' or 'I don't feel like having sex now.'"

Slowly, however, attitudes are changing. "[Ali Kagashe's] are obsolete ideas, ideas of the 18th century," says Dr Christian Mukoyogo of the Faculty of Law at the University of Dar es Salaam. Women also have their right of choice." According to Anna Mgongolwa, who also lives in Dar es Salaam, "Such people are a stumbling block in the way of women's liberation. They are not only obsolete in ideas and deeds but also insensitive to natural changes and evolution." Younger people tend to agree. "Gone are the days when a girl had no rights to anything. Today a girl and a boy are at par," says 21-year-old George

Kengo, who works with the Tanzania Railways Corporation.

Gradually, it appears, Tanzanian men, particularly those who are educated, are beginning to accept women's sexual needs. "If he forces her, he is being unfair to her. A husband or a man worth his salt has to agree to justifiable reasons advanced by his partner as to why she is not ready for sex," considers Dr Paul Senge of the National AIDS Control Programme. Pharmacist Denis Chuku says that "a wife and husband should agree that it is time for sex. This kind of agreement wards off any possibility of resentment on the part of the wife or denial of her rights in the course of sexual intercourse." The same approach, he says, should apply outside marriage.

The power of tradition

Among the traditional customs that still hold sway, particularly in rural areas, are female circumcision and widow inheritance, both of which play a role in transmission of HIV.

Female circumcision – known as female genital mutilation by those who oppose the practice – is still common and is often performed crudely by individuals with no medical training. Peter Mwera, who works for the Save the Children Fund in Tarime, says that 5,000 girls a year in the region are circumcised, 20 of whom die during the process. The survivors risk childbirth complications due to inelastic scar tissue and a variety of other health problems. Furthermore, HIV may be transmitted by the use of unhygienic knives. "We have identified some girls, and boys, who already show signs of HIV symptoms and we suspect that circumcision has done the harm," says Mwera.

Widow inheritance occurs when a man dies and a brother or close relative undertakes to look after his surviving wife; by having sex with him, the woman indicates that she has accepted him as her new husband. Where a man has died of AIDS, his wife is likely to have contracted the virus. In such cases, she may deny or be ignorant about the risk of transmitting the virus to the man who inherits her. Dr A

Mtango of People in the Struggle Against AIDS in Tanzania (WAMATA) recounts an incident in which a widow would not admit that her husband had died of AIDS. She conceived a child with her new partner, who already had two wives – presumably placing them all at risk. Yet for the woman, who had no other source of income, there appeared to be no alternative than to persist with her denial.

The practice of widow inheritance is slowly dying away. "It is not easy to eliminate a custom that has persisted in a culture for so long, but the best approach is to take an HIV test before the inheritance is carried out," argues Dr George Sangiwa of the Muhimbili Medical Centre in the capital. He concedes that testing is likely to remain a rarity in rural areas because of poverty, distance from testing facilities and adherence to tradition.

Men need sex

Within the framework of traditional life there is significant scope for men and, to a lesser extent, women to enjoy sexual relations. Indeed, many people believe that sexual abstinence is harmful for both men and women and can cause skin rashes and other symptoms.

While men are supposed to have sex only with their wife or wives, they nevertheless justify sexual activity before and outside marriage. Young men, for example, believe they must have regular sex. Kali Ali, who is 19, says that a man has to have sex and any woman can satisfy his sexual needs. James Rwabwisho, a 27-year-old resident of Dar es Salaam, has a slightly different approach: "Women differ. You need to taste a variety of them to get varied magnitude of enjoyment. Some are sweeter than others."

Marriage provides a sexual outlet and the opportunity to become a father. "I do have sex to get children to inherit me, pleasure notwithstanding," says John Kalungo. Older men have sex for the same reasons, although less frequently. Paul

Bachuleka, 61, from Muleba district, 69-year-old Musa Bilali from Dar es Salaam and 59-year-old David Gawaza of Muleba town all confess that sexual urge and power diminish with advancing years. "I was able to go four or five rounds in one night when I was young. Nowadays I only manage one round a month," says Bilali with a laugh.

Lack of children or the desire for more provides one rationale for extramarital sex, but other reasons are also given. "Those men who are not satisfied look for women outside because they want more 'trips' than their wives can endure," says Catherine Bugya from Kanyigo village in Bukoba rural district. Bugya adds that most women lose their sexual desire after having children as they get more attention and love from the children than from their husband. The implication of her remarks are that men's continuing sexual desire justifies sex with other women.

In some rural communities, a wife returns to her parents during pregnancy and childbirth. "A wife knows that her husband will definitely run with other women during her absence, and society knows it, though it doesn't openly sanction it," observes radio journalist Clement Mshana. Furthermore, "some cultures believe that once a child has been delivered, she has to leave her husband alone until the child reaches a certain age, for fear that having sex will seriously affect the child. This creates a loophole for a husband."

Older men often seek sexual contact with young women, who are considered disease-free, easy to satisfy economically and with the potential to revitalise ageing partners. "I am 46 years old. When I make love to a young girl of 18 I feel born anew – leave alone the psychological satisfaction," says a man sipping beer in a Muleba township bar. In such circumstances, he adds, it is easy to forget the existence of AIDS. Others might point out that forgetting the existence of AIDS makes it more likely that his young partner will contract the disease from him than vice versa.

Women too

Women are also recognised as having sexual needs. A wife has cause to complain if a husband denies her intercourse. "It is common in some tribes for a woman to pack her things and leave for her parents' home because of denial of her sexual rights. She goes back after her husband has settled the difference with her in front of her parents and other distinguished elders," says Halima Khatibu, a District Commissioner in Mwanza, in the north-west.

A husband is never offended if his wife initiates sex, says Dar es Salaam butcher Bakari Ali. Fortunata Shayo, a clerk in Dar es Salaam, agrees that women also need sex. "It is a question of tuning oneself," she notes. "Some women tune themselves when their partners are away. They forget about sex and the urge disappears. But some women can't tune themselves and have to have regular sex, otherwise they get backaches or become mentally disturbed."

Miriam, a 20-year-old civil servant, is unusually outspoken when complaining about her boyfriend. "Recently I tried to get another man who is heavily built and goes the long distance," she says, with none of the shyness that other women show when talking of such matters, "yet he doesn't satisfy me."

Women in cities have greater sexual freedom than their rural counterparts. "Lack of higher education makes village husbands conservative, and this affects the freedom of their wives," says Fidelis Silas of the charity World Vision in Muleba district.

Catherine Bugya points out that some wives seek revenge when they discover their husband going out with other women. Comments Janet Kabwela of Muleba district: "Lack of mutual trust prompts husbands to go out to have sex. Some wives, though not as sexually free as men, will secretly do the same for revenge." If women put up with their husband's unfaithfulness, "their meekness puts them at a disadvantage." But not all women are meek. "If you are

Sexual Practice

Tanzanians have a variety of methods of increasing sexual pleasure. In Kagera region, arousal may be achieved by drumming the clitoris with the penis. This practice, known as *katerero* and enjoyed by both sexes, leads to 'wet sex' – copious vaginal secretion – and helps women reach several orgasms. However, as the regional AIDS Control Coordinator Dr Mussa Ndyeshobora points out, **katerero** often results in skin abrasions that facilitate HIV transmission. *Katerero* is also seen as incompatible with condom use. Women who feel they do not secrete enough vaginal fluid to please their partner may seek herbal treatment that may itself cause injuries that facilitate the transmission of HIV.

In other areas, men prefer dry sex – little or no vaginal secretion – because, they say, their partners feel like virgins. "A loose, wet vagina is a sign that a woman has had lots of sexual partners," believes Peter, a 41-year-old civil servant. To please their men, therefore, some women insert herbs, powders or pastes into their vaginas to make them dry and tight, although it makes intercourse difficult and unpleasant. "When I am dry, I get vaginal ruptures which cause severe pains. I get pains for a week," complains a woman from Dar es Salaam. The insertion of herbs and friction during intercourse are likely to cause abrasions that increase the risk of HIV transmission.

Little research has been undertaken into the impact of *katerero* or dry sex on transmission of the disease. A survey in Mwanza region showed that bruising during sex was reported by more men (23 percent) than women (10 percent), though this was not associated with dry sex. The survey also revealed that 10 percent of those questioned were aware of anal sex, but the extent of the practice is unknown [2]. ∎

married, you should not tolerate your husband or wife having sexual affairs. You can find yourself unconsciously chopping off his male organ, which is the source of the problem," says Marthe Kavishe, 31, a housewife in Dar es Salaam.

Now and then

Tanzanian women are far more likely than men to meet their sexual needs within marriage. In studies of rural and urban adults in the north of the country [3], 15-25 percent of women and 49-53 percent of men reported having casual sex. Six percent of men and 27 percent of women reported only ever having one sexual partner, and 28 percent of men and only two percent of women reported more than 20 sexual partners in their lifetime. While married and unmarried men were equally likely to have more than one sexual partner, married women were less likely than unmarried women to do so. Men are also more likely to have pre-marital sexual experience; most women questioned married within two years of losing their virginity, while a majority of men did not marry until six years later. By the age of 24, 97 percent of women had married, compared to only 56 percent of men.

It is unclear whether pre-marital sex has become more common in recent years. In one of the surveys, in 1993 in Mwanza region [4], 66 percent of women over 45 but only 39 percent of women under 24 had sex before their 16th birthday, suggesting a rise in the age of women's first intercourse. For men, 46 percent also said they began their sexual lives before 16, but the percentage has not changed over the last few decades. However, a 1989 survey in rural areas of the North Mara region [5] suggested that the age of first intercourse was static amongst women (half the respondents had lost their virginity by their 15th birthday) and falling amongst men (half of men over 40 had their first sex before their 17th birthday, and half the under-19s had lost their virginity by the time they were 14).

Whether true or not, every generation believes that morality was more strictly observed in the past. So it is not surprising that people believe unmarried men and women today are more sexually active than were their parents or grandparents. Goreth Bisibe, 38, says, "Girls and boys no longer hide but do openly what was until recently considered taboo."

Sixteen-year-old Agnes Alphonce of Buganguzi village in Muleba district offers a perspective common among young people: "There is a lot of sex. A girl and a boy will meet sexually not once, not twice, but many times. Youth in schools as well as in villages engage in pre-marital sex with their fellow youths and adults." She adds that adolescents are ridiculed by their peers if they do not have girlfriends or boyfriends.

Money talks

Education and wealth also affect people's risk of contracting HIV, but they affect men and women differently. The more educated a woman, the more likely it is that she will have only one sexual partner [6], while, as in other parts of sub-Saharan Africa [7], educated men are more likely to have several partners. Wealth has a similar impact: the poorer a woman and the wealthier a man, the more likely is each to have several sexual partners.

The impact of poverty on a woman's sexual behaviour begins when she is young. While young men engage in pre-marital sex to prove their manhood, points out Dr Stephen Katende of the African Medical Research Foundation (AMREF), girls between 10 and 15 commonly seek men willing to pay a small fee in return for sex. Pancras Kyeju, a teacher in Kagera, says that "as long as parents are unable to buy necessary items for their children, the children will always look for an alternative way. If a girl doesn't get enough money from her parents while at school, she will definitely have sex to get money for cosmetics, clothes, modern shoes and so on." When older men are not available, according to one report, "schoolboys provide their female classmates with gifts such as exercise books, pencils, bars of soap or cash in the range of Tsh 50-500 [less than US$1.00] in exchange for sex" [8].

Mariam, now 17, remembers the first time she had sex. She was 15 and the man was her father's age. "I didn't like it as my private parts were still small and I felt great pain," she recalls. "But I needed money to buy new shoes and new clothes for Eid [a Muslim festival] celebrations. My parents were too poor to afford them." She became pregnant and had an abortion. "The man paid the bill and has since forgotten me. But I learnt the trick and now I don't worry about getting pregnant. I can 'skin' any man without fear," she says – but she refuses to discuss HIV.

Godeliva Mashamda, 18, from Muleba district, claims that student girls "are easily tempted by simple valuables like shoes. They use any means to get things which their parents cannot afford to provide." Georgia Kalaze of WAMATA points to the effect of men from the city visiting their home villages: "Once rural girls and women see these men, they rush to them in the hope of getting money or a chance of being chosen as life partners and taken to towns where they believe life is a paradise."

Women's limited chances of achieving financial independence underpin the economic pressures for sexual barter. "I had better die of AIDS rather than starve to death," says Asha, a 23-year-old sex worker in Dar es Salaam. Her perception is similar to that of Agnes in Muleba: "Some people are afraid of AIDS. If it kills us, then we die like other people have died," she comments fatalistically, adding that she will not starve as long as men are available. Not all women share her attitude. Julieth Ndumbalo, 36, who sells buns to sustain herself and her two-year-old daughter, says no man forces a girl or woman to have sex: "They make themselves loose in order to get money and live a luxurious life."

Protection

The fact that relations between men and women in Tanzania allow sex to occur in many different situations renders both sexes vulnerable to HIV. Health education programmes emphasise mutual faithfulness and abstinence as primary means of preventing HIV transmission, but many people regard these methods as unrealistic. At least one study indicates that awareness of HIV/AIDS does not necessarily lead to self-protection, particularly amongst men, although women with good knowledge of AIDS are likely to have fewer sexual partners than women whose knowledge is poor [9]. Nevertheless, over a two-year period the proportion of men reporting sex with more than one partner fell in Mwanza from 22 percent to 12 percent [10].

"High awareness of [male] condoms has not apparently led to widespread and appropriate use," says James Kakoba of AMREF. Kakoba blames this on many factors, including "inadequate education on the use of condoms, poor access, especially for people in the rural areas, high costs, poor distribution and emotional constraints." Others point out that various religious denominations strongly oppose their use.

In one survey only one in five respondents said they had ever used a condom and only one in 10 used one the last time they had intercourse [11]. In that and another survey no more than 34 percent of men questioned and 14 percent of women had experience of condoms [12], and a third study has seen no significant rise in their use [13]. On the positive side, condoms may be used by many of those who are most at risk, who have more than one sexual partner and who have sex under the influence of alcohol, as well as those with higher levels of education [14].

Many people object to condoms. Bus driver Shaban Rajab claims that "condoms are not safe. They put the AIDS virus in them and that is why I don't use them." Others are concerned about out-of-date condoms, fear that condoms do not really provide a barrier against HIV, or believe that a wrongly worn condom can cause friction and burst. "A condom can be retained inside a woman, thus necessitating medical intervention for removal," says Jane, 24, who works in a guesthouse in Bukoba town. Still others claim condoms reduce sexual pleasure. "With a condom on you do not feel the sweetness very well," says a married man in Muleba town.

Cultural values often hinder their use, since buying condoms is synonymous with talking openly about sex. "Condoms are not displayed openly in rural areas. People have to ask for them covertly, often using veiled terms like 'sell me a weapon'," says 19-year-old Switbert Andrew. Andrew adds that if a man cannot afford a condom or cannot find one to buy, he goes ahead without it.

Many women feel too shy to insist on their use. "I can't afford to tell my boyfriend to use a condom as this amounts to saying that I am a prostitute. Further, when my partner puts on a condom, I know that once he ejaculates I won't feel the ecstasy of the action," says Adelina, 26 (though experts agree that it is physiologically impossible for a woman to feel a man ejaculating inside her). Adelina notes that a woman has to be careful not to make her financial supporter angry, a point acknowledged by many others, women and men.

Masturbation

Although mentioned by some health promotion programmes, masturbation is not widely promoted as a means of releasing sexual tension. Indeed, the practice is often seen as a kind of weakness. "If one fails to get a lover, the notion of masturbation doesn't come very quickly as very few people prefer it. Some people believe that those who prefer masturbation are mentally disturbed and others believe that the method reduces man's sexual performance," say Anthony Ruta and Gosbert Kakele, from Kishanda village in Muleba district.

"It reduces both the man's and woman's sexual desire and people who practise masturbation are mentally disturbed, experience body fatigue and lose much sperm," considers Sotery Christian, a retired primary school teacher in Kabulala village in Muleba district. When asked to resort to masturbation instead of risking AIDS by not using a condom, one man in Muleba responded, "I had better do without sex.

Sexual starvation does not kill, but [masturbation] injures and can make somebody crazy. Do you think I'm crazy enough to masturbate?"

Signs of change

The overall picture may be unclear, but there are signs of change, particularly amongst the younger generation. Young men are more likely to listen to women who want to use condoms or who refuse to have sex. "Never without a condom. If my partner is not ready for it, he had better pack and go," says Jamillah Juma, a secretary in Dar es Salaam. Furthermore, education and stronger political will could overcome many of the obstacles to partner reduction and condom use.

Others point out that one way to check the spread of HIV/AIDS is economic development, with an emphasis on vulnerable groups. "There is a need for income-generating possibilities for women and young people in order to improve their relative strength in the community and minimise their need for sexual bartering," says Hadija Riyami, a senior journalist with the government-owned *Daily News*. Health education activities could also be stepped up, including AIDS information points in villages and greater availability of condoms. More information on condom use, safety and disposal and reassurance that they do not hinder pleasure would increase their acceptability among both urban and rural populations. Such drives are not happening because of limited funds.

It is axiomatic that men's respect for women is essential in defeating HIV/AIDS. As Dr Roland Swai of the National AIDS Control Programme points out, there is a woman behind every success in any endeavour carried out by a man: "AIDS will be defeated only if men respect the views and advice of women, who are the most vulnerable group in this case."

THE SOUL IS WILLING

INTRODUCTION

The religious impulse is common to all humanity. Belief in a god or gods has motivated human behaviour since pre-history, and the moral standards in each society reflect the standards we believe the deity or deities have set for us. Whichever religion comes closest to universal truth, few of us claim complete awareness of the deity's wishes. We depend on interpretations of holy writings and sayings, interpretations by individuals like ourselves who can interpret religion only within the limits of their culture, their intelligence and their empathy for other human beings.

Perhaps nowhere has religion – at least the monotheism of Judaism, Christianity and Islam – come into greater conflict with human behaviour than over the question of sex. Most religions exhort celibacy until marriage and fidelity thereafter, but no society has ever achieved such an ideal. Indeed, many religious leaders fail the morality that they preach, and television evangelists in the United States, preachers in Africa and monks in Asia are revealed to have committed adultery or broken vows of celibacy. Religious followers are equally human: Muslim countries such as Bangladesh have high rates of sexually transmitted disease while Italy, the heart of the Roman Catholic faith that bans contraception, has one of the lowest birthrates in the world.

Anathema or God's love

This conflict between ideals and reality and varying interpretations of dogma allow different religious responses to HIV/AIDS. Some religious leaders insist that all prevention must be based on celibacy and mutual fidelity, while others recognise that we all lead imperfect lives. For the former group, condoms are anathema; for the latter, to promote condoms is to express God's love.

Joyce Djaeleni Gordon, who works in HIV prevention in Indonesia, suggests one way of overcoming religious leaders' insistence on an ideal that many people find impossible: "I take groups of nuns and priests in everyday clothes, as well as Muslim leaders, to red-light districts in order to observe. They are never the same after a field trip. All of a sudden, everyone in the street becomes real and they begin to see the subtle nuances of the people involved in prostitution, rather than just seeing things in black and white." The main difficulty, Gordon goes on, is in persuading those of higher ecclesiastical rank to come on these journeys of discovery. Nevertheless, the outcome is that HIV prevention workers "may never get a stamp of approval from the 'institution' of religion, but religious leaders will not stand in the way of prevention efforts once they understand the whole picture"[1].

In fact, religious leaders in many countries have become active in HIV prevention with an approach that is more pragmatic than dogmatic. The Archbishop of São Paulo has been quoted as saying that while he cannot accept condoms for the prevention of life (that is, as contraception), he is in favour of condoms for the prevention of death (to prevent the transmission of HIV). In Thailand monks run workshops for children in temple schools and make visits to the homes of people living with the virus.

Men, women and faith

Most religious leaders are men and it is reasonable to question whether their interpretations of scriptures, consciously or not, disadvantage women. Certainly, as described below, the Bible and Koran imply that men have authority over women. Nevertheless, fierce debate continues in many churches over the role of women as priests, while Muslim feminists argue that "it is not the religion but the male interpretation of the Koran that keeps women oppressed" [2].

In Ghana almost every citizen professes a desire to obey God's commandments. Not surprisingly, the conflicts between sex and faith and over the relative status of men and women form part of the ongoing debate as to how the community as a whole and individual believers should respond to a disease that affects more than one in 50 of the adult population. Mike Anane's report does not argue whether one response to HIV/AIDS is closer to religious ideals than another, but it does provide an insight into the response of spiritual leaders to the epidemic. There are disagreements with secular authorities, but these are benign in comparison with the brief portrait painted by Eda Chávez of the conflict in Mexico between church and state.

RELIGION, MEN AND HIV/AIDS IN GHANA

by Mike Anane

"I told my mother about it when I read a love letter which I found in my husband's pocket and realised that he was seeing other women. She asked me to have patience and go back to him, since that is how men behave. When I told my friends in the church, they asked me not to tell anyone since in view of my position [in the church] there would be a scandal if people learned that I have left my husband because he is flirting. They advised me to continue to stay with him and pray for him to change his behaviour. But here I am now doomed forever…"

The 35-year-old lay Christian preacher and mother of three sobs as she tells her story. She has been diagnosed HIV-positive after several weeks of incurable diarrhoea and fever. Her 38-year-old husband, a well-to-do businessman, also has the virus and admits having sex with other women. Three of them, including an 18-year-old girl still at senior secondary school, also have the virus.

The situation is not unusual. A strong belief in God is integral to most Ghanaians' lives but this has not prevented more than two percent of the adult population from contracting HIV. Women are particularly badly affected, representing 70 percent of those who have fallen ill or died from the disease and 80 percent of those between the ages of 15 and 30 living with the virus. As women are affected, so too are children: 50,000 are believed to have lost one or both parents to AIDS, a number that is expected to rise to 150,000 by the year 2000.

Three of every four Ghanaians belong to a Christian denomination, while 20 percent of the population are Muslims mostly living in the north of the country. The rest of the population practise traditional African religions or minority faiths such as Buddhism.

Despite the overwhelming numbers, the Reverend Amoako Andoh of the Christian Council hesitates to call Ghana a Christian society, preferring the description 'pluralistic'. Certainly, the churches play an important part in community life and are uniquely placed to influence attitudes and educate large numbers of people about HIV/AIDS and sexuality. Indeed, many church leaders have exhorted Ghanaians to respect the commandments of no sex before or outside marriage, but many people, it seems, have not heard the message, disagree with its contents or find the injunctions impossible to uphold.

"We are helpmates; no one is the driver"

Both the Bible and the Koran appear to accord women secondary status to men. "Wives, submit to your husbands as to the Lord, for a husband has authority over his wife just as Christ has authority over the church"* [3]... "Men are the protectors and maintainers of women, because Allah has given the one more strength than the other, and because they support them from their means" [4]. But both scriptures also assert the need for mutual respect between the sexes.

---

* Translations from the scriptures in this chapter are intended as guides only.

Pastor Samson Azubike of the Berea Christian Faith Ministry comments, "There is no doubt the Bible says women are subordinate to their husbands, but the same Bible says 'Husbands, love your wives just as Christ loved the church and gave his life for it'" [5]. The Reverend Amoah Kumah of Kwashieman Presbyterian Church adds that men are given the privilege of head of the community, but that privilege should be exercised only with love. Hajia Ketumeh Mahamah, president of the Federation of Muslim Women's Associations, points to the Koranic description of marriage for her interpretation of equality between the sexes: "They are your garments and you are their garments" [6].

Yet the fact that their religion urges mutual respect between the sexes is forgotten by many Christians and Muslims, and there is frequently a discrepancy between scriptural teachings on relations between the sexes and the way that many people, particularly men, interpret those teachings. Many believers, men and women, consider that a woman's first duty is to be a helpmate to her husband, regardless of his behaviour. As a result, Kumah sees women as imprisoned by false notions of what they can or cannot do, while Mahamah recognises that "some Muslim societies have never regarded men and women as equals in marriage."

Sex and marriage

Both religions believe that God created sex to bring fulfilment to husband and wife. Because marriage is, in Christian terminology, a sacrament, sex itself is a sacred act. Out of respect for that sacrament, men and women should be chaste before they wed and faithful to their spouses thereafter. Pre-marital sex is therefore condemned by St Paul, who tells Christians "it is better to marry than to burn with passion" [7], while the Hadith (the sayings and traditions of the Prophet Mohammed) says, "A young man who can take care of a household should marry, but if you cannot, then resort to fasting to dampen the sexual urge" [8].

Both religions condemn adultery. The Bible's Book of Proverbs asks: "Can you carry fire against your chest without burning your clothes? Can you walk on hot coals without burning your feet? It is just as dangerous to sleep with another man's wife. Whoever does it will suffer" [9]. The Koran warns believers that adultery is an abomination and an evil, and that adulterers should be stoned to death [10].

The religions differ in their attitude to polygyny, forbidden by the major Christian denominations but permitted in Islam. The Koran urges: "If you can, marry of the virtuous women one or two or three" [11]. Many people interpret this attitude as recognition that men's sexual needs are greater than women's, but according to Ahmed Dery of the Muslim Family Counselling Services, "To avoid prostitution involving women whose husbands had died from the various Islamic wars, men were allowed to marry more than one." He explains further that, at least theoretically, polygyny in no way implies lack of respect between the sexes: "A man can only take a second or third wife if his first wife/wives agree, and if he has the financial resources to take care of them and he can treat all his wives equally."

Mahamah emphasises the notion of equality between the sexes, pointing out that Koranic legislation protects the rights of women in marriage, child custody and inheritance. "The intent of the laws of inheritance was to give all members of a family a share and women in particular financial autonomy and security." However, she says, many Muslim girls marry unaware that they can negotiate the terms of the contract. "If women knew the rights Islam has given them, they would be able to question the man, refer him to the Hadith and he would pay attention."

The soul is willing, but...

The commandments of church and mosque may be clear, but not all Ghanaians abide by their rules, even when they wish to. As Ekow, a 33-year-old banker, puts it: "As a child I was very obedient to the teachings but these days I can no longer control myself. I think the sex drive is overwhelming. It hasn't therefore been easy to stay away from pre-marital sex."

Samuel, 42, a lawyer, thinks his soul is willing but his body is weak. "I regret it each time I indulge in extra-marital sex and I ask for forgiveness; it's the temptation of Satan." Elsie, a 26-year-old secretary, discloses that financial difficulties sometimes drive her to sleeping with men. "I know God does not like that but I need the money to look after my bed-ridden mother and my younger brother."

Others claim they adhere to the church's teachings, although it takes determination. Vivian, a 28-year-old teacher, "used to be very promiscuous even though I was going to church regularly, until one day I surrendered my life to Christ and started praying every day for a renewed lifestyle. So in my bid to please God I am no longer promiscuous." Kofi, a 45-year-old truck driver, used to "continue with my sexual pranks and pray each time for forgiveness." Now, however, "I have been able to put a stop to my negative activities."

Muslim men find it equally difficult to live according to their religion. Tahiru, who has two wives, prays five times a day, "but for me this has become a formality, so the concentration is not there. I am always in a hurry to finish praying, more so when it is Friday and my girlfriend is waiting for me." Seidu comments that it is difficult to be a Muslim in a country where Muslim law is not applied. "Every day I walk the streets and I meet women who are almost naked [that is, wearing miniskirts]... The temptation is always there for me and it is proving hard to resist every day."

Of wives and concubines

The discrepancy between religious teachings and the practice of believers places women at a disadvantage and, as the statistics demonstrate, makes them particularly vulnerable to HIV. One AIDS prevention worker points out that men and women are trapped by religious conventions requiring women's subservience, which makes them vulnerable to infection. Even when a woman knows that her husband has been unfaithful and may be HIV-positive, she considers it her duty to have sex with him.

Women appear more likely to abstain from extra-marital sex than men. Pastor Samson Azubike suggests this is the result of different attitudes towards the consequences of sexual behaviour. "Men think they have nothing to lose but women think of what could happen: the chances of not getting married in future if she has a record of pre-marital sex, pregnancy, and danger in abortions." Also, Azubike points out, precedents encourage some men to have sex with many women: "Some religious leaders have numerous wives and concubines because they believe they are following the traditions of respected biblical figures such as Abraham, Solomon and David."

Reverend Kumah of the Christian Council recognises that many women have contracted HIV partly because they are physically more vulnerable to the disease and partly because of the struggle to survive. "In Ghana, as in other parts of Africa, many women have no sources of income and they must survive, no matter the cost. That is why some of them give themselves to men and damn the consequences."

Dr Cynthia Eledu, UNAIDS country programme advisor, points out that it is not only men who are unfaithful; some older men marry younger women but cannot meet their sexual needs, leaving the women to seek solace elsewhere.

Hajia Mahamah agrees that the discrepancies between ideals and practice place women at risk. "The Koran is particularly solicitous about women's welfare and development but it is no secret that this is not what prevails in Muslim communities." Furthermore, Mahamah believes that polygyny can exacerbate the problem of a woman's inability to ask her husband to use a condom if she depends on him economically and is in competition with his other wives. "A lot depends on the level of education of the women involved, since educated and enlightened women in such relationships are more independent and more likely to behave differently."

Polygyny in itself is not a risk factor. As Dr Lawson Ahadzie, former coordinator of the National HIV/AIDS Control Programme, points out, it is fidelity rather than the number of wives that is important. "Who is practising risky behaviour: the acclaimed polygamist who has three or four wives and sleeps with them alone or the unacclaimed polygamist with four or five concubines who sleeps with all of them including his wife?"

A curse from God

Although HIV is widespread, many religious leaders are reluctant to address the issue. Some priests refuse to discuss AIDS in their sermons because they believe it is the result of immoral behaviour and a curse from God. Others have been reluctant to bury people who have died from the disease or to provide pastoral care for patients with AIDS. Some clergy insist that couples take HIV tests before any formal marriage ceremonies can be performed in church. Reverend Godfried Bamfo of the Christian Council says this is because "we do not want to marry any infected persons." Other religious leaders appear to agree that a test is desirable but are uncertain as to whether the couple should not marry if one or both tests positive.

Dr Kweku Yeboah, director of the National AIDS Control Programme, is against the idea of compulsory tests. "I believe the couple themselves should decide that they want to know each other's status, then the two agree. Assuming one of the couple is positive, what will the church do about it? Does it have the right to say they should not marry?" Yeboah warns that even if the couple test negative, there is no guarantee that they will never contract HIV, because it is "your later life that determines whether you will get infected or not."

Religious leaders and believers are divided over the 'cause' of AIDS. Cynthia, a 50-year-old retired midwife, is convinced that the disease is a curse from God. Pointing out that "the person suffering from the full-blown disease grows extremely lean, and all flesh and muscles are eaten away," she claims that severe loss of weight is described in the Book of Proverbs [12] as the punishment for adultery. Some people with AIDS share her view. Kojo, 40, says: "Traditionally, when you incur the wrath of the gods and they pronounce a curse on you, your body is consumed by a strange disease with strange symptoms, almost a mixture of any disease. AIDS is no different."

Pastor Dickson Sarpong Tuffour of the Central Gospel Church claims that HIV comes not from God, "who loves us", but from the devil. Reverend Amoah Kumah has a view closer to that of the epidemiologists, blaming the epidemic on such factors as the breakdown of family structures, infidelity in marriage, sexual activity among the young and lack of reverence for the value of life.

Whatever the views of individual clerics, most denominations recognise that people living with HIV require support. As Pastor Azubike points out, "St Mark's Gospel is replete with cases of Jesus showing compassion to sick people rejected by society." The church's prominent role places it in a unique position to offer community-based assistance for families affected by the disease. For example, outreach programmes managed by the Catholic church include the Nkawkaw Holy Family Diocese in eastern Ghana, which has programmes in weaving, pillow-making and other handicrafts for people with HIV/AIDS.

Yes to abstinence, a qualified no to condoms

Most churches believe that HIV/AIDS prevention is best promoted through God's teachings of abstinence before marriage and fidelity afterwards. In the words of Reverend Bamfo, "No sex before marriage; no sex outside marriage – Best Vaccine against HIV/AIDS."

Before AIDS, many Christian denominations discouraged or banned condoms on the grounds that God's first commandment to humanity was "Be fruitful and multiply" [13]. However, some churches now accept condoms within marriage for family planning purposes, although few recommend them as a general means of preventing the spread of HIV.

Reverend Kumah explains why: "There are so many ways of doing this: behaviour change, abstinence, condom use for married couples. The moment you promote condoms it's as though you are trying to say that promiscuity is OK!" Kumah adds that condoms can break, and extends his disapproval to the female condom, which he sees as encouraging women's promiscuity. "Men may go on trek, they travel for days. Women would feel free to do whatever they like and this is where the problem lies with the female condom." Other religious leaders express similar opinions: "We are not saying, Do not use the condom," says Bamfo. "We are saying, The condom is not the answer. The answer is to live with Christian values or return to our cultural values."

Some church leaders appear a little more accepting of condoms. Dr Ralph Avornyo, AIDS control coordinator of the Catholic Secretariat, states: "The Catholic church would not counsel the use of condoms when one married partner was unfaithful because it is not the duty of the Catholic church to tell him or her to use the condom. However, we shall expose them to all the preventive methods and if they choose the condom, it is their choice."

"Passports to Death"

Lack of money, conservative attitudes, machismo and, above all, the opposition of the Catholic church to government and non-governmental information messages have placed serious obstacles in the path of efforts to combat HIV/AIDS in Mexico.

In a country where 90 percent of the population is Roman Catholic, the church has a strong influence, which it exercises directly and through wealthy private organisations. In recent years the church has stepped up its campaign against condoms, using a range of arguments including xenophobia and supposed scientific data suggesting that latex does not prevent HIV transmission.

Archbishop Norberto Rivera Carrera claims that "it has been proved that contraceptives cause emotional and psychological damage in women and, in the case of condoms, are another artificial method of preventing the conception of life." Rivera Carrera suggests that the message 'harmful to health' should be included with every condom. In response to the government's anti-AIDS campaign, launched in mid-1997, the group Pro-vida (For Life) launched a court action against the Ministry of Health, accusing it of instigating "genocide" by its promotion of a "useless ... and dangerous instrument". Other declarations have described condoms as "passports to death".

The church has also played the nationalist card, claiming that campaigns promoting condoms reflect the interests of multinational manufacturers. "These laboratories fill their pockets with money at the cost of the immorality of the population encouraged to libertinage." The church has also alleged that campaigns are imposed by imperialist interests in the First World – a culture "traditionally uninterested in birth". In yet another argument the pastoral secretary of health of the Mexican Catholic church explains that Mexican men find it difficult to adapt to the use of condoms because "they are not in the national mentality", while conservative groups have claimed that condoms have "a power greater than hormones for awakening the libido".

Conflicting messages from the government and church have sown confusion in some minds. Laura Rosales, a 34-year-old housewife, is typical of many when she admits, "I don't know what to think." However, the church's campaign may have been counter-productive in some cases, with leading figures, such as the rector of the National Autonomous University of Mexico and the director of the National Polytechnic Institute, declaring themselves in favour of condoms as a prevention measure. ∎

Eda Chávez

Both Bamfo and Avornyo are hostile to widespread promotion of condoms. "Do not let us tempt children with sex and condoms," says Bamfo. "What they need is discipline and self-control." Avornyo laments, "The way we are showing condoms on television is bad. Children are buying condoms and experimenting." Such an attitude is shared by many lay Christians. Cynthia, the retired midwife quoted earlier, believes that as long as condoms are promoted as offering complete protection against the transmission of HIV, "sexual promiscuity and infidelity will never end."

Many Muslims accept condom use within marriage. Ahmed Dery of the Muslim Family Counselling Services states that "at our last sensitisation meeting [in 1997] for Muslim leaders there was consensus over the need for protection, but of course no one will come into the open and say the youth should use condoms. The problem comes when condoms are being used by unmarried couples, and our religion does not permit that." Hajia Mahamah claims that "the present media promotion of condoms is working against us." She cites the instance of a TV commercial in which a young girl's mother asks whether she has her condoms when she leaves the house. "What are we teaching these children?" she asks.

"Prevention is the only way"

Some religious organisations have implemented prevention programmes. The Scripture Union's 'AID for AIDS; Design for the Family' project promotes Christian and traditional moral values within a strong family life. In the words of Reverend Bamfo, coordinator of the project, "AIDS has no cure, so prevention is the only way." The Catholic church has founded Youth Alive clubs in schools to drum home the need for abstinence. In addition to four health clinics, the Christian Council has community-based distributors who advise on AIDS and birth control. The Council also has a day-care centre at Ho in the Volta region; Reverend Kumah explains: "Initially, it was not easy getting parents to talk, so this nursery was built as a bait. Now we can talk to parents about family planning and AIDS."

To spread skills on reproductive health issues and HIV/AIDS, the Planned Parenthood Association of Ghana (PPAG) organises courses for instructors from a range of Christian and Muslim associations. The trainers are expected to conduct a series of workshops and seminars to sensitise their respective audiences on HIV/AIDS.

Some churches go further than education. Aware that many impoverished young women in the Volta region travel to neighbouring countries to practise prostitution, a Catholic organisation at Agomanya has set up a ceramics factory and is developing a bakery with the 31st December Women's Movement, with the aim of developing a source of income for members.

Are men different?

Some religious leaders believe they should work differently with men because men are more likely than women to have sex outside marriage. Others are of the opinion that preaching God's word is enough. Reverend Joseph Amponsah of the Calvary Baptist church says, "We emphasise that men are the heads of their families and have the responsibility of leading the rest of the family to learn about the work of God ... we tell them also to lead exemplary lives worth emulating."

Pastor Ato Wilson of Central Gospel Church says, "This male problem needs to be addressed seriously by the church. The message is that men are at a greater risk." Reverend Edwin Donkor discloses that his church is forming a men's group to discuss issues particularly relevant for men. He adds, "We already have a women's group and we counsel them so that they are aware of all the tricks that men are up to."

However, Major Mrs Marlene Jones of the Salvation Army insists that anti-AIDS campaign activities in the church should not necessarily target men. "It is not what you are but what you do," she counsels. "If there is any group that we should target, it is the women, for after all they give in to the men and we must teach them to say no and also other ways to prevent the disease."

HIV/AIDS workers respond

Many HIV/AIDS prevention and health workers criticise the church's insistence that condoms should be used only within marriage or not at all. Alex Banful of the Ghana Social Marketing Foundation, which promotes condoms across the country, argues that, "Abstinence is the ideal. But while you're preaching abstinence you should protect people before they get the message about abstinence." Professor Fred Sai, an AIDS expert, points out: "Religious leaders have been preaching abstinence etc for generations and it has not worked." Marian Amissah of the Ministry of Health adds: "It's fine to pray for God to help you abstain but we must also not forget that the condom can be a saviour when some temptations prove too hard to overcome."

There are many examples of unmarried men and women who are unwilling or unable to abstain from sex and who need to be persuaded to use condoms. Sai cites "youngsters in the streets fending for themselves who are easy prey to all sorts of people", while Banful points to the high rate of teenage pregnancy in Ghana, an indication that many young people have sex without birth control. Napoleon Graham, head of research at the Planned Parenthood Association of Ghana, argues that condom use demonstrates responsibility. "When a young man comes here to buy condoms do we say, 'He is not married so we will not sell to him'?" he asks. "Wouldn't it be better to sell to him for protection than let him go and do it without any protection?"

Banful is the strongest critic of the church leaders' stance. "Religion is the biggest problem we have. It is encouraging women to give in to their husbands any time they ask for sex, instead of encouraging spousal communication, which would enable women to ask their husbands to use condoms when they believe he is seeing other women." Other HIV/AIDS prevention workers are less critical, arguing that the church and the mosque have done good work in terms of prevention and care.

Cynthia Eledu of UNAIDS says, "Religious organisations have been around longer than HIV/AIDS and they have chalked up some successes in the prevention of the spread and transmission of certain sexually transmitted diseases. Their teachings, messages, morals and behaviour can provide the strong motivation that old and young people need to avoid the danger of HIV/AIDS." Marian Amissah of the Ministry of Health adds that it is important to involve religious leaders in the anti-HIV/AIDS campaign because the population at large trusts information that comes from them.

A yawning gap

The spread of HIV in Ghana, as elsewhere, is alarming. There is a yawning gap between the religious beliefs that most Ghanaians profess and the sexual lives they practise. Each year thousands of men fall into this gap and thousands of women are dragged in with them. Surely religious leaders have a duty to construct a bridge of tolerance by recognising that many people are unable to live up to the ideals of chastity and mutual fidelity, and that condoms play a valuable role in saving people's lives. Furthermore, religious leaders, who are mostly men themselves, need to recognise the extent to which HIV is spread by men's behaviour against the will of women.

FROM BOYS TO MEN

INTRODUCTION

The onset of puberty brings with it the capacity and desire for sexual experience but not the knowledge to use that capability wisely. In many cultures in the past, public ceremony marked the transition from child to adult and appropriate sexual behaviour was learnt in private. Sometimes this education was formal, as a relative took charge of the child's instruction; sometimes it was informal, through casual remarks and banter in single-sex groups. In some societies a girl heard that respectable women displayed no pleasure in sex, while in others she was taught how to please her partner and to demonstrate that he pleased her. Boys usually learned haphazardly, often gleaning little more than that they should 'prove' themselves with many sexual partners.

When puberty rites marked the boundary between childhood and adulthood, the concept of adolescence was unknown [1]. Today, however, as millions of young people find themselves physically mature but not yet accorded the rights and responsibilities of adults, the term 'adolescent' becomes relevant worldwide. Furthermore, the skills and knowledge appropriate to traditional cultures are no longer adequate in a world of loosening community bonds, frequent migration and widespread Western influence. Traditional knowledge often masks ignorance, which leads to unwanted pregnancies and high rates of sexually transmitted infections (STIs). If present and future generations are to be protected from the undesirable consequences of sexual behaviour, new skills and knowledge must be taught.

Sex education

There are strong arguments for early and universal sex education. Twenty percent of the world's population – 1,200 million people – are aged between 10 and 19. Each year 60 million boys and 60 million girls reach sexual maturity and must be convinced of the need to protect themselves and their partners. By current reckoning, at least four million will contract HIV at some point in their lives. It is not only adolescents who are at risk; many children begin sexual activity, voluntarily or under compulsion, before puberty [2].

While it cannot protect against violent abuse, appropriate sex education can help young people understand the implications of sexual activity and develop the skills to refuse it if they wish. Where adolescents are ignorant of sexual matters there are often high rates of sexually transmitted diseases and teenage pregnancies; where adolescents have access to sex education they tend to delay having sex, have fewer partners and are less likely to conceive or contract sexually transmitted infections [3].

Sex education is usually taught in schools, partly to reach as many young people as possible and partly because parents and adolescents are often uncomfortable discussing sexual matters with each other [4]. When parents do discuss sex, it may cause more problems than it solves: "The image of sex that [Ugandan parents] portrayed was a very negative one, giving rise to instructions which are not explained in any way, such as, 'If you want to die, go and see the boys/girls'"[5].

As this report shows, sex education must encompass more than the mechanics of intercourse, contraception and disease prevention. Young children should learn what behaviour is acceptable for both children and adults and how to refuse inappropriate advances; older children need a description of the physical and other changes that will take place as they enter adolescence. Before sexual activity begins, all young people should be aware of the consequences of intercourse, in addition to knowing how to refuse sex and how to ensure that sex they undertake is safe.

The format of sex education will vary according to culture and the age and sex of the participants. One project in Zimbabwe noted that both boys and girls in their early teens were willing to talk about sexual and relationship issues, while slightly older girls were reluctant, perhaps because they "had already begun sexual activity and did not want to incriminate themselves through something they would say." The oldest girls, however, were more confident and more willing to enter into discussions. The same project noted that mixed-sex sessions "encourage debate and sharing of ideas [and] allow children to learn from and appreciate each other," but certain topics, such as puberty, care of one's body and the reproductive system, were best discussed in single-sex sessions [6].

Sex education should also include sex between men and between women. Although attitudes towards this form of sex include hostility and disdain, many young people have experience with partners of the same sex and some are at risk of contracting HIV through this route. For example, 25 percent of one group of Sri Lankan young men and adolescent boys reported sex with another male, with nine percent having experienced anal intercourse [7].

Boys and girls

Sex education helps young people make intelligent choices, but it is a relatively new discipline and even the best devised programmes do not always meet the needs of their audience. One study of condom promotion in Denmark, for example, points out that sex education often begins by teaching the mechanics of reproduction, which then leads to questions of love, pleasure and self-identity, whereas young men's sexual experience begins with self-identity, moves on to seeking pleasure and love, and only later comes to the question of reproduction [8].

The Danish study underlines the point that boys and girls have different expectations and needs that extend beyond understanding their own bodies. Furthermore, sex can have very different consequences for male and female adolescents. Young women bear the most direct consequences of pregnancy, including the decision of whether or not to abort. As Latin American researchers point out, "Very few adolescent boys require hospital admission for health problems related to sexual behaviour, while pregnancy-related causes represent the bulk of hospitalisations for young women"[9]. And although both sexes are prone to sexually transmitted infections, young men are more likely to seek treatment, since young women may be unaware that they have contracted potentially serious infections.

In general, therefore, male adolescents tend to want frequent intercourse and pay little attention to possible pregnancy, while female adolescents are expected to decline sex and to fear pregnancy. As discussed earlier, the result may be that early intercourse is a much more positive experience for young men than for young women. Appropriate sex education is a means of redressing at least some of that imbalance.

Life skills in Uganda

While most governments pay lip-service to the idea of protecting children and adolescents from HIV/AIDS, few have thrown their weight behind comprehensive and nationwide sex education. One exception is Uganda, which in the late 1980s emerged from almost two decades of dictatorship and civil war to find itself in the midst of one of the world's worst AIDS epidemics.

To assist national recovery and development, the incoming civilian government made it a priority to introduce Life Skills Education in every school, a key component of which is sex education and the skills to avoid unwanted sexual activity. Other institutions in Uganda, including non-governmental organisations (NGOs) and the media, have also become involved in informing young people of the many issues surrounding sexual behaviour. This is no easy task, particularly because many adults, including teachers, are themselves uncertain of the facts about intercourse and appropriate sexual behaviour.

Nevertheless, despite considerable obstacles, the impact of such a policy is clear. Many boys, and no doubt girls, continue to believe that men must have intercourse, but condoms are now widely accepted and, it appears, widely used. As a result of this intensive, government-backed effort, Uganda has progressed from being one of the countries worst affected by HIV to one of the few in which rates of infection appear to be falling.

MALE ADOLESCENCE AND SEX EDUCATION IN UGANDA
by Ogen Kevin Aliro & Henry MK Ochieng
with Anne Akia Fiedler, Editor of Straight Talk

"Sex education for boys in my day? Not in my tribe at least!" Thirty-year-old Eddie Ejalu, a member of the Iteso tribe from Pallisa district, 200 kilometres east of Kampala, the capital of Uganda, expresses his surprise at the idea. "It was taboo to discuss sex in Teso. To mention a word describing the genitals amounts to a shameful abomination. They call it *akiro nuka ileic* – something shameful," he says.

Ejalu's reaction is typical. For generations of Ugandans, whichever of the nation's 60 tribes or ethnic groups they belonged to, there was no open discussion of sexual issues. In some tribes young girls learned, usually from an aunt, how to please their future husbands while their brothers learned from uncles and older boys that sexual prowess was a sign of manhood. That was the limit of sex education. In other ethnic groups, such as the Iteso, young men and women got their first ideas about sex from gossip in peer groups. Relatives played no part in the process, except when a mother cautioned her son not to spend long nights out, as was the custom during Ejalu's pre-marital days.

Traditional attitudes

Although civil war and urbanisation have radically altered lifestyles in recent years, traditional attitudes are still influential throughout Uganda. While there are differences between the tribes in the forms of sexual behaviour considered appropriate for men and women, there are nevertheless many similarities across the nation.. Men are expected to 'perform' – to have frequent sexual intercourse with one or more partners – and women are expected to remain faithful to their husbands and to please them sexually. It is impolite to discuss sexual matters in public, except among other members of the same sex; even then the tone is more likely to be jocular or boastful and there is little opportunity for serious discussion.

Almost every culture marks the transition from child to adult, although here too tradition is under threat. At adolescence among the Iteso, Jop'Adhola and Acholi tribes, for example, girls move into one big house while each boy has his own small hut. Every second year the Gishu circumcise all boys who have reached the age of 16. (Because of HIV/AIDS, a fresh blade is used for each initiate, whereas in the past a single blade was used for all participants in a ceremony.) However, this change in status is seldom accompanied by accurate information on sex, conception or the risk of disease.

"Do not lie in bed like a log"

The five million Baganda comprise the largest ethnic group. Like the neighbouring Banyoro and some other tribes, they formally educate young women on how to be good wives. At a very young age a girl receives some information on sex from her mother, but when she reaches nine years old her *ssenga* (paternal aunt) takes charge, taking her out of the village to the privacy of the bush, where she is given intensive instruction in sexual matters.

"Your aunt explains that when you get married you are supposed to please your husband sexually. For instance, you are told not to lie in bed like a log," says Sarah Sembatya, a young Ganda woman. In similar approaches by other groups, a range of advice is passed on. The Ankole, for example, a pastoral tribe in the south-west, tell girls that the cure for insufficient release of vaginal fluids is to drink plenty of yoghurt.

In a number of cultures, including the Baganda and Banyoro, young women are not only expected to know how to please their men, but to modify their bodies for them as well. Girls practise *kusika*, methodically pulling and stretching the *labia minora* and clitoris every day for a month or more. The idea is that the elongated lips curl themselves around the man's penis during copulation, heightening his pleasure. Sometimes herbs are used to assist the process. Among the Ankole, where a girl's virginity is highly prized, *ebikooza* aids the pulling while *ekyomoro* heals the wounds that develop in extending the labia. Even today in many cultures, girls are expected to 'pull', although the disruption of traditional family communities through war, urbanisation and boarding schools has undermined the practice in many areas.

In urban areas, where many children attend church-run schools, sex education for girls was equally limited. According to Juliet Mulindwa, who grew up in the 1980s, "We were taught mostly about hygiene, how we must take care of our bodies during our monthly cycles, but there was never any education about condom use or sex. When we got out of school we just picked knowledge from here and there." Mulindwa adds that many of her friends shrouded sex in mystery. "Some of them called it a fun-filled dirty act. The subject of sex was a taboo, hence the secrecy."

"Your uncles encourage you to find a girlfriend"

While Ganda girls were receiving formal instruction from their aunts, their brothers learned about sex from their older peers. There was no formal instruction process, according to 25-year-old Mark Sserunkuma.

In many cultures boys were expected somehow to know about sex, and put that knowledge into practice. Omwony Ojwok, the AIDS Commission Director-General, remembers that among the Acholi Labwor in the north a boy's father would become anxious if his son never brought girls home. And while there was uproar if an unmarried girl became pregnant, boys were encouraged by their peers and fathers to get girlfriends to prove they were 'real' men and not impotent.

Among the large Acholi tribe, long famed as warriors, there was even stronger encouragement for boys to prove themselves men. Komakech Lagira, 23, says that once an Acholi boy reached 14 and moved into his own *manyatta* (hut), "you were warned against closely associating with your sisters as this could 'spoil' you. Then you were discouraged from spending your evenings at home. Your parents would start wondering and worrying if you rarely went out at dusk."

Lagori adds, "In Acholi there isn't any direct teaching about sex but your uncles would keep encouraging you to get a girlfriend." However, times are changing. Acholi culture has been destroyed by the vicious insurgency which continues to ravage northern Uganda, while AIDS has levied a heavy toll and brought hitherto unknown worries about uncontrolled sexual relations. "Most youth now proceed with caution," Lagori says.

Among the Ankole, according to James Tumuheirwe, "The boys never got any specific lessons. You were expected to learn from your uncles' tales as nephews and uncles wandered the plains grazing the family herds. That is the time you learned about how to handle girls and what happens in marriage." He adds: "Your dad would be a very happy man if he noticed that you had started spending nights out."

Before the circumcision ceremony among the Gishu, a boy's maternal uncles give him lectures on his 'new' life as a man, but this covers social more than sexual behaviour. Mike Wadada, himself recently circumcised, explains that he learned how to treat his future wife and how to behave in the company of his in-laws. "For example, they will explain you aren't supposed to come into contact with your mother-in-law," he says, a custom common to many of the country's tribes and ethnic groups.

The window of hope

In 1986 the new civilian government headed by Yoweri Museveni inherited a country devastated by war and AIDS. More than a decade later the war has ended but the epidemic continues to exact its toll. According to UNAIDS, almost two million people in a population of 20 million are believed to have died from the disease, 1.7 million children have lost one or both parents to the epidemic and more than 900,000 adults and children currently live with the virus.

If there is any means of slowing or halting the epidemic, it lies in what experts such as Professor John Rwomushana, head of research in the Uganda AIDS Commission, call 'The Window of Hope': children between the ages of five and 14. Few at that age are HIV-positive: babies who contract the virus from their mother usually die young and adolescent sexual liaisons generally start after 14. It is, however, a narrow window. Rwomushana points out that the age group with the highest rate of HIV infection is the 14- to 25-year-olds, with girls under 19 six times more likely to have contracted the virus than boys of the same age.

Into the 21st century

The first attempt to introduce sex education for young Ugandans was made in the late 1980s. HIV/AIDS prevention messages were included in the Life Skills Education Initiative developed as part of the School Health Education Project (SHEP), inaugurated by the government and the United Nations Children's Fund (UNICEF) in 1985. The target audience was primary school pupils aged 12 or 13, although the programme was later extended to younger children. The upper age group was chosen because most had not yet started sexual activity and it was considered particularly important to educate girls before they dropped out of school to start families, a risk which increased from 14 onwards.

However, when SHEP was assessed it was discovered that although children were aware of health issues, their behaviour had not changed. According to educator Joy Oguttu, "Children had a lot of theoretical knowledge about health but lacked the basic skills to apply it." To overcome these difficulties, in 1995 the government, with the support of UNICEF, launched BECCAD (Basic Education, Child Care and Adolescent Development Intervention) with the publication of *Into the 21st Century: Life Skills Education Resource Booklet.*

For use in primary and secondary schools, this teacher's manual defines life skills as the "personal and social skills required for young people to function confidently and competently with themselves, with other people and in the wider community". Such skills were formerly taught by families and communities, but "traditional methods have largely broken down, thereby leaving children much more vulnerable."

Topics covered by the programme include hygiene, self-esteem, inter-personal communication and environmental preservation, as well as health issues such as smoking, alcohol, sexually transmitted infections (STIs) and AIDS. The last includes the social factors that lead young men and women to have sex.

Men and women

As Jolly Zamukunda of the Ministry of Education and Sports points out, BECCAD programmes emphasise gender issues, specifically promoting equal standards for boys and girls. "It challenges both boys and girls to be responsible and is aimed at empowering both sexes."

BECCAD does not formally challenge traditional beliefs, such as the idea that boys' education is more important than girls'; that women should do all the household chores; that girls, but not boys, should be virgins on marriage. But it encourages children and teenagers to consider these issues. As the manual states, "Girls should not be looked upon as sex objects. They are individuals like any male, have ambitions, dreams and goals which they should pursue."

BECCAD does not give answers, but encourages pupils to work out answers for themselves. For example, an exercise describes a head prefect (the top boy in a school) telling a girl how much he likes her. Pupils are asked to describe what might happen next and to consider such questions as, "Is love shown by having sex?", "What skills does one need to ensure that one does not have sex until s/he is ready?", "What skills do boys need to respect a girl who says 'no'?"

Straight Talk

While BECCAD ensures that some aspects of sex are discussed in school, perhaps the most important initiative for young people is *Straight Talk*, a magazine on sexual and related issues targeted at literate urban youth. Every month 95,000 copies are printed, 35,000 of which are distributed as an insert in the state-owned daily newspaper *The New Vision*. An additional 21,000 go to 69 NGOs working throughout Uganda, 18,000 are sent to more than 900 secondary schools and 7,000 go to tertiary (further) education institutes. The remaining copies are sent to churches, medical institutions and *Straight Talk* clubs that have been formed by young people specifically to receive and discuss issues in the paper. *Straight Talk* began as a source of information about HIV/AIDS but has evolved into a magazine that covers all aspects of reproductive health, including emotions and attitudes. It reinforces the message that love is not sex and that boys as well as girls can control their sexual desires. One column is committed to debunking myths – explaining, for instance, that the hymen does not harden and the penis does not shrink if sex is delayed, and that a girl can conceive during her first intercourse.

Safe sex is still an integral part of the magazine. In a recent issue the doctor warned that relying on "'safe days' to prevent pregnancy is very risky; because adolescent girls don't ovulate or menstruate regularly, it's almost impossible to predict which days are safe." He added, "...and of course, there are no 'safe days' from HIV/AIDS! On any day of the month you can get an STD including HIV." Other HIV-related issues, such as the vulnerability of women under 18 due to the immaturity of their vaginal tract, have also been covered.

The only topic which the magazine has avoided – in the belief that society was not ready to discuss it – is sex between men or between women. However, when doctors and counsellors from the magazine visit schools, it is a subject which students always want to discuss, and the editorial team now intend covering it.

Shared experience

Straight Talk encourages readers' participation, both through its letters page and through its question and answer section. Some questions are common to both boys and girls, such as whether sexual abstinence leads to sterility, when is the right time to start having sex and how to use condoms properly. But many girls want to know about lasting love and maintaining a relationship without sex, while boys are more concerned about how soon they can have sex and the size of their penis.

Comments in a recent issue of *Straight Talk* included, "I have never had sex with any girl, although I make friends with them. I spend some of my free time with my grandfather's tortoise. I advise the youth to avoid being idle because it is a source of evil." Another young man from Kampala wrote, "Before I started reading *Straight Talk*, my motto was: 'Anything in a skirt, no sparing.' I have come to realise that I was buying nails for my coffin. My motto for 1998 is, 'No-sex is not a disease; and no condom, no sex.' Reader, follow it." A third commented: "If you are afraid of having sex with your girlfriend, it means that you are not ready yet."

Straight Talk has been outspoken in advocating masturbation for both sexes as a way of avoiding unwanted consequences of sex. Readers have been advised on pleasurable ways of masturbating, such as not rubbing too hard and using a little oil. Many letters tell of masturbatory experiences. A typical comment comes from a boy who wonders if three times a day is too much; the counsellor's advice is that if the reader thinks it is too much, he should think critically about why he is doing it.

Are boys listening?

Increased openness about sexual matters was also evidenced in a conversation with nine Kampala boys in the 17-20 age group.

Ben and Robert believe boys should start having sex at the age of 12, because, Ben says, that is when they begin to produce sperm, "and this should be released during sex." Donald and Adam agree on 15 because, according to Adam, "it is at this time that boys learn what is right and wrong." Andrew suggests 16, "because they are in the middle of adolescence and can control themselves a little bit." Only three of the group suggest 18. That is the age when a boy becomes a man, in Kalungi's view, and at which emotional maturity begins, according to

Khamis. Kavuma favours 18 because of the threat of AIDS: "The earlier you start, the shorter your lifespan." Most believe that young men should have sex before marriage, because it is too difficult not to or because it is important to gain experience "so they don't mess up when they get married."

The boys' attitudes towards girls' wishes is contradictory. All agree that a girl who does not want sex should be "respected and left alone", yet all claim that when a girl says 'no' she means 'yes', and half of them have strategies for trying to get a girl to change her mind. "I persuade her with more sweet words to agree to have sex with me," says Kalungi. "I become extra nice to her and try to take off her clothes," says Moses. As for married women, only Ben thinks that they should always have sex when their husband demands it, but three of them believe that, if a wife refuses, a husband has the right to have sex with other women.

All the boys agree that condoms are important for the avoidance of pregnancy and disease, "which can interrupt studies", but several offer rationalisations for failure to use a condom. Adam, for example, says condoms are not needed "if a girl is a virgin and does not want to use condoms and if both partners are sure they are safe and want to have children." Ben claims that a boy need not use condoms if they cause pain to his partner (an unlikely occurrence).

In a discussion with a similar group of girls, aged 15-19, all report that boys try to pressure them into sex, and those who have started sexual activity claim that they always use condoms. They say persuading boyfriends to use condoms is not a problem, as long as the request is made at the beginning of the relationship.

A step forward

As the quotes above confirm, boys' attitudes towards women have changed only a little. "Sex is used as a means to prove manhood and is regarded as a vital part of a relationship, without which it is bound to break up," says Dr Sarah Naikoba of the Naguru Teenage Health and Information

Centre in Kampala. "Boys are under pressure to practise in order to become 'perfect' lovers and lack of sexual prowess is a sign of failure as a man."

Because "most boys believe that women are physically weak, they can never have equal rights with men in relationships," she observes.

Nevertheless, Naikoba sees some hope. "Urban boys have more positive attitudes towards women than their rural counterparts. This is because the urban boy is more exposed to independent women, whereas in rural communities most women still depend on men for decisions."

In addition, a decline in the incidence of sexually transmitted diseases in many areas, reported in a Ministry of Health HIV/AIDS report in March 1997, has been attributed to increased condom use, and Naikoba says some boys would not be shocked to find a condom in their girlfriend's bag. This suggests that condoms are now an integral part of many Ugandans' sexual lives – which is definitely a step forward.

A DOUBLE LIFE

INTRODUCTION

Worldwide, 10 percent or more cases of HIV infection may be the result of sex between men, [*] *and the actual total may be much higher. It is not clear why most men prefer women sexually and some prefer men, but male-male sex has occurred in every known society and at every recorded period of history [1]. Where societies have differed has been in the extent to which such behaviour is accepted or persecuted by the majority.*

The concepts of 'homosexual' and 'gay' are widespread only in Western culture and in segments of other societies influenced by the West. 'Homosexual' describes men and women who prefer sexual relations with their own sex (as 'heterosexual' describes men and women who prefer relations with the opposite sex). 'Gay' refers to homosexuals who seek legal and social acceptance of the right to live with a partner of the same sex.

Elsewhere sexual identity is often defined differently. In Latin America it is generally defined by penetration – machos insert; women and maricones (effeminate men) receive. In South Asia 'real' sex is between a man and a woman and results in children, while sex between men is seen as play, as described below.

Such definitions can be broken down further. Partly reflecting Western influence, in one group of 17 men who have sex with men in Madras, India, eight called themselves danga or kothi (feminine men who are penetrated), two panthi (men who only penetrate), three 'double deckers' (men who penetrate or are

---

[*] As elsewhere in this book, references to 'men' include adolescent boys who have reached sexual maturity.

---

*penetrated), two 'bisexual', one 'gay' and one 'homosexual' [2].
In Costa Rica, as explained in a later chapter, a man who has sex
with men may be a 'topman', 'chicken' or 'possum', while a
Peruvian man in the same situation may be a* mostacero,
cacanero, activo, maricón, cabro *or* resquete, *depending on his
social status and perceived sexual role [3].*

*Indeed, as suggested elsewhere in this book, a man's sexual
identity often depends at least in part on his age, marital status and
economic power: that identity may change according to the situation
in which he finds himself and the partner with whom he has sex.
(The picture is further complicated in societies which recognise a
third gender or transgenders, such as* travestis *in Brazil or* hijras *in
India.)*

*Sexual identities reflect perception as much as reality. In private
a macho may be penetrated by a maricón, and an Indian man may
consider sex with his male partner of greater importance than sex
with his wife. Where taboos against sex between men are strong, a
dichotomy may arise between sexual* identity *and sexual* activity,
*as when a man who usually has sex with other men nonetheless
considers himself heterosexual. Sometimes the dichotomy between
identity and activity is so strong that whole societies deny that sex
between men occurs, or they insist, as in parts of Africa and Asia,
that it occurs only amongst those who are 'degenerate' or have been
influenced by foreign cultures.*

Desire and behaviour

*Not only does identity sometimes differ from activity, but desire can
differ from behaviour. Like women, some men have sexual relations
against their will with partners they do not want. Men who prefer
men but who are afraid to defy society's taboos may spend a lifetime
as husbands and fathers, while some men in single-sex institutions,
such as prison or boarding school, have sex with other men
voluntarily or through coercion, even though they prefer women.*

*Furthermore, behaviour and desire may be unrelated. As
described earlier, discharge rather than pleasure may be the goal of
sex and opportunities for discharge may occur frequently. In India,*

"There is social acceptance of males sharing beds, of male to male affectionalism, both in public and private. This often means that a significant amount of sexual behaviour occurs in family environments, between uncles and nephews, cousins, friends and even at times brothers. This is not seen as real sex. It is maasti. *Sex is between a husband and wife!"[4]*

Given these differences between desire and behaviour [5] and between activity and identity, and the widespread reluctance to admit to same-sex behaviour, it is difficult to estimate how many men have sex with men in different cultures across the world. Recent surveys of male bisexual behaviour range from (national or regional statistics) 0.5 to three percent in Mexico and three percent in Norway to five percent in Brazil, 10 to 14 percent in the United States, 15 percent in Botswana and Peru and six to 16 percent in Thailand [6]. Even if the details of these studies are open to dispute, the overall conclusion can be drawn that men who have sex with men are found in every society and at all levels of social and economic life.

It is also clear that men who have sex with men are not an isolated group. Most also have sexual relations with women, for a short period or throughout their lives, although they may not describe their relationships in the words of this young Trinidadian man: "I had this wonderful relationship with this lovely young lady. At the time, I had a male lover. She pretty much accepted it because she knew I was gay; I was kind of like her trophy. For me it was exciting because it was a new experience and she was beautiful and I really enjoyed it."

Preventing transmission of HIV

Unprotected anal intercourse has the highest risk of sexual transmission of HIV – and omitting this fact from education campaigns may actually increase the incidence of anal intercourse between men and with women. A 1996 Panos study revealed that in many countries and cultures there is still little or no recognition of the existence or the extent of sexual activity between men, and the response of governments in particular has been non-existent or minimal [7]. This means that the extent to which sex between men is a significant factor in the AIDS epidemic is uncertain, and that in some countries assumptions of an exclusively or predominantly male-female epidemic need to be re-examined.

In the English-speaking Caribbean, health authorities are looking again at the role of sexual transmission between men, prompted by awareness that many men are reluctant to admit sexual activity with other men and by the high percentage of cases in which transmission is reported as 'unknown' – 18 percent across the region and as high as 35 percent in some countries. Dr Bilali Camara of the Caribbean Epidemiology Centre points out that "in countries where [sex between men] is most accepted, we see that there are less cases of 'unknown'." The implication is that many of these 'unknowns' are in fact attributable to sex between men. A similar analysis may be valid in Mexico, as discussed earlier in this book.

Camara suggests that social pressures on men who prefer men may be perpetuating the epidemic in the Caribbean. "If society is really pushing people to be married and does not tolerate homosexuality, we will be battling for a long time." He adds that only when society as a whole accepts that some men prefer sex with men will it be possible to "empower people to accept what they are and do the correct thing – that is, practise protective behaviour." Indeed, where male-male sex is taboo and the opportunities for men to establish sexual relationships with each other are severely curtailed, the result may be more frequent partner change and therefore more opportunities for HIV transmission.

The Kenyan experience

While sex between men is accepted in very few societies, over the last 20 years there has been increasing awareness that it occurs all over the world. Community organisations for men who are to a greater or lesser extent open about their attraction to other men have been founded in countries as disparate as Zimbabwe, Bangladesh and Japan, while bars, cafés and bathhouses that cater to this clientele can be found in large cities everywhere from

Buenos Aires to Beijing. Often the emergence of specifically gay organisations in developing countries can be traced to the need to respond to the HIV/AIDS epidemic [8].

In sub-Saharan Africa, as in many Muslim countries, there is still widespread reluctance to recognise the phenomenon, although the subject is gradually coming under scrutiny across the continent. In addition to widespread controversy in Zambia and Zimbabwe, coverage has included a version of this article published in mid-1998 in The Nation *in Kenya and an interview with a homosexual man published in the Ivory Coast magazine* Infos *in February of the same year.*

The following report by Wanjira Kiama [9] opens a window onto the lives of Kenyan men who have sex with men. As one of the first, if not the *first, study of men who lead 'a double life' in that country, it provides important insights into a phenomenon that even now continues to be denied by many Kenyans. It cannot, however, be comprehensive, and the following points should be noted.*

Firstly, the fact that the men interviewed live in Mombasa and Nairobi does not mean that sexual activity between men is restricted to these cities. As in every country, the relative anonymity provided by cities allows greater opportunity for sex between men, but men who have or wish to have sex with men are to be found across Kenya and across Africa. Secondly, the men Kiama interviews are relatively open about their sexual activity and many have obviously thought carefully about the conflict between their desires and prevailing Kenyan customs. Others who were not interviewed and who are less open about their sexual activity would describe their situation very differently; many would consider themselves 'men' or 'heterosexual' and reject any identification as homosexual or gay.

Thirdly, Kiama's suggestion that sex between men is more tolerated in Mombasa because of Arabic influence may be true, but, as the article suggests, the activity itself occurs irrespective of cultural or tribal influence. Finally, for many of those interviewed the ultimate goal is a strong emotional relationship – love – with another man, and sexual activity is a means of both expressing and searching for that love. This is not to deny that many sexual acts between men in Kenya and elsewhere are simply a desire for physical pleasure and relief.

MEN WHO HAVE SEX WITH MEN IN KENYA

by Wanjira Kiama

"I would rather sire a cow"

Jomo Kenyatta, Kenya's first President, once claimed that there is no African word for homosexuality [10]. This proves, he argued, that homosexuality is foreign and totally un-African. According to Daniel arap Moi, the current President, "Kenya has no room or time for homosexuals and lesbians. Homosexuality is against African norms and traditions, and even in religion it is considered a great sin" [11].

Kenyatta's and Moi's opinions reflect a disapproval that runs broad and deep in Kenyan society. Typical is the attitude of Michael Kariuki, a 37-year-old accountant with a non-governmental HIV/AIDS organisation. "Homosexuals are a menace to society. They should not only be jailed, but the key to the lock should be thrown away," he says heatedly. Asked what he would do if he learned that his son was homosexual, his anger rises: "I would disown him before I caused him grievous harm. I would rather sire a cow than a homosexual. With a cow you get milk, but what possible good or value would come out of a homosexual?"

In Mombasa, on the coast, there is greater acknowledgement of homosexuality, but little more acceptance. Men who are believed to have sex with men are despised, ridiculed, harassed and sometimes beaten during political campaigns – emotionally charged periods when people commonly express deep-seated fears and hatreds – and often threatened with lynching.

Children shout *shoga* (male prostitute) at them in the streets.

This hostility reflects generally conservative attitudes in society towards all aspects of sexual behaviour. Despite one of the severest HIV/AIDS epidemics in the world, government officials have removed from the school curriculum any subject, topic or learning material that touches on sex education, including *Family Life*, a booklet published by the American Girl Guides Association. In August 1995 the Roman Catholic Archbishop of Nairobi joined hands with the Imam of Jamia Mosque, Ali Shree, as they led their faithful in the burning of condoms and sex education books in a Nairobi public park.

Kenyan law defines any sexual relations between men as a criminal act. There have been few prosecutions, but in early 1998 police began an investigation into FOPOGAP (Forum for Positive Generation on AIDS Prevention), a registered community organisation for people with HIV in the western town of Kisumu. Police alleged that the organisation was 'recruiting' homosexuals.

An unknown quantity

The rarity of prosecutions is no doubt one of the factors behind Attorney-General Amos Wako's statement that his office does not know the extent of homosexual practices in the country. Wako repeats the government's line that homosexuality is widely regarded as un-African and that the wider public does not see the need for research in this area.

"What we have on this is just impressions, since there are no reliable figures anywhere," says Dr Frank Njenga, a consultant psychiatrist who is chairman of the Kenya Medical Association's social responsibility committee and an HIV/AIDS prevention activist. "People tend to either exaggerate or underrate the extent of homosexuality, bisexuality and lesbianism." Njenga argues that Kenyan society has not reached the point at which people with a different sexual orientation are allowed to be themselves or develop within a set of laws and rights set out for them. As a result, "we have a good number of Kenyan men who are constitutionally homosexual and socially heterosexual, so as to fit in society."

The only national statistic relating to homosexual activity is the informal UNAIDS estimate that fewer than five percent of AIDS cases are the result of sexual transmission of HIV between men. Studies by AMREF (the African Medical Research Foundation) of the high incidence of sexually transmitted diseases among truck drivers plying their trade between Mombasa and Uganda show some evidence of homosexual activity, particularly with boys aged 12 to 16. "It is not known whether it is men expressing their own sexuality, or whether it is something learned," says Dr. John Nduba, deputy director of AMREF's Kenya office.

Such studies are supported by anecdotal evidence that suggests sexual activity between men in Kenya is more common than generally believed. Young people, usually men with men and women with women, often share housing for economic reasons. According to Allan Ragi, coordinator of the Kenya AIDS NGO Consortium, however, some young men share housing for emotional and physical needs. He adds that, although not officially acknowledged, homosexuality is practised in prisons, the military, boarding schools and colleges throughout the country.

Ragi claims that more young men than old participate in homosexual activity. An anonymous AIDS programme manager with an international NGO agrees: "Men having sex with men is not only common amongst young people, but fashionable. Just as young men like to wear an earring, they are also opting to try out homosexual practice. It is not just seen as an orientation, but also a 'fancy lifestyle'."

According to interviews with men who have sex with men, the most common sexual activity is anal penetration. Roles within a relationship are often clearly defined, with the same partners taking the active (insertive) and passive (receptive) role. Those who are looking for steady relationships often do not rush into sex, preferring to get to know each other well first. In such situations the relationship progresses from appreciative looks to touching, kissing and cuddling, before more intimate touching and finally to sexual intercourse. Those who are interested in casual relationships want only sex, sometimes watching erotic videos to put themselves and their partners in the mood.

Due in part to the constraints on relationships between men, a good number of those interviewed have intense, short-lived relationships. Sometimes men give up relationships with other men, either to see if they can be happy in relationships with women or, under pressure from society's reaction to men who have sex with men, to practise celibacy.

A national phenomenon

Statistics on men who have sex with men may be difficult to obtain, but the men themselves are to be found across the nation. Kisumu, for example, has a reputation for homosexual activity, with men such as gardeners, cooks, hotel staff and shop attendants having relations with their – usually older – employers. According to a man familiar with sexual practices in the region, money rather than desire appears to be the motive for many of the younger men, while the older men have the wealth to conceal their lifestyle from public scrutiny.

Perhaps not surprisingly, it is easiest to find men who have sex with men in the capital, Nairobi, although not everyone is aware of this. Paul, a 39-year-old technician with the University of Nairobi, married with three children, convulses with laughter when asked whether he knows any homosexuals. "What would I be doing with homosexuals? Don't I look man enough?" he bellows. Yet within walking distance of the university, in a building open to the public, young men who openly refer to themselves as gay meet on a regular basis to socialise. A few come for a 'sun-downer' (a drink at the end of the day) wearing make-up and jewellery.

Others are more discreet. Odongo, for example, 42, is a petrol attendant who grew up in Kisumu and pays for male partners. His family forced him to marry, but he has no sexual relations with his wife, who still resides in Kisumu. Jared, 55, from Luoland in western Kenya, works as a casino manager and owns a big house in an affluent Nairobi suburb. He has been married three times and has a six-year-old daughter. All his wives left him after finding out that their marriage was just a front. Jared goes to church every Sunday "to pray for my sin", but is unable to abandon his lifestyle.

Amin, 54, is a primary school headmaster with a double life: a public life during the day, and another every evening in the backstreets of Nairobi. He consumes *miraa* (a form of cannabis) in a bar-restaurant where he can drink, eat and pick up young men; he will take his new partner to a more private establishment where he can hire a room for sex before driving home to sleep. His relationships are with men in their twenties, whom he assists financially and not all of whom are homosexual.

Peter, a 50-year-old property developer, once married and now divorced, is seen frequently at social functions with different young women. When the party is over he escorts the women home, then takes up his male relationships in private.

Men who have sex with men are perhaps more accepted in the coastal regions of Kenya, where the Arabic past heavily influences the Swahili culture. There is a Swahili word for homosexuality (*msenge*), and marriages between men. At 23, Hassan, for example, has been married three times, complete with dowry and wedding rings. Hassan appears very feminine, pouting his lips and covering his face when laughing. He walks with a swing while holding his *kanzu* (robe) under his arm, the way some women carry themselves. He wishes his marriages had been legal, so that he could claim his rights from the husbands who abandoned him. He believes that one in particular, whose parents forced him to take a wife, will return. "I used to cook for this man, make his bed, and be there for him. Yet he left me," Hassan says in deep sorrow.

Just as older women, known as *mkungus*, educate young girls in the duties of marriage, on the Kenyan coast young homosexual men learn from male *mkungus*. Ahmed, 36, who lives in Mombasa, learnt bedroom tactics from a *mkungu*, as well as how to groom himself, to deal with diseases and to keep his man happy by being a good cook. The training lasts a month. At the end the younger man gives the *mkungu* special cloth and kitchen utensils as payment. Ahmed is now a *mkungu* himself, advising on perfumes that will please the 'husband' and demonstrating how to wear the special *khanga* (flowered cloth) in the house. "You must be clean and smell nice to your husband all the time," he tells his disciples.

For eight years Karim, 30, who also lives in Mombasa, has maintained a relationship with the 40-year-old man married to his cousin. Five years ago the cousin caught them in bed. To hush things up Karim was asked to marry his lover's 16-year-old adopted daughter. From Karim's point of view it was a good arrangement, as it offered him the respectability of a wife as well as continued access to his lover, now his father-in-law. With no experience of women, on his wedding night Karim forced himself to provide his relatives with the evidence that he had broken his wife's virginity. He has a five-year-old daughter but does not want another child. On two evenings a week he and his lover hire a hotel room, where they spend several hours before returning to their wives.

At the travel agency where he works, Karim's colleagues know he is gay. The women are friendly. Some men despise him, others approach him in private. Karim believes that most men in Mombasa enjoy sex with other men and rejects the theory that homosexuality was brought in by tourists. Fazal, 30, a mechanical engineer with an 18-year-old lover, agrees. Now faithful to his partner, as a teenager he had several experiences with fellow boys. "Many men in Mombasa try out homosexuality in their youth," he says.

Abdul, also 30, is a businessman who travels frequently to

the Gulf. He was a virgin when his parents arranged a wife for him, and they have a two-year-old daughter. But for three years Abdul has been in a relationship with another man his own age. They have a small flat in which they meet regularly and where Abdul does all the housework. In his own house, where his wife and sisters prepare and serve his food, the roles are reversed.

Rocky, 23, comes from western Kenya and was brought up in Mombasa. He is a language student who hopes to become a tour guide. When he was younger a neighbour his father's age introduced him to homosexual activity. Their affair lasted three years. For the moment Rocky does not have a stable relationship. "Marriage is not an option for me," he says. "God made me and understands me. I don't think what I do is a sin."

In the closet

Most men who have sex with men in Kenya do not admit their secret to family members or even to close friends. The pressures of leading a double life can be acute. Abdul appears to adore his male lover of the last three years, but says that now he has a one-year-old son he is tired of "playing the woman". He would like to begin a new life and stop his homosexual relationship. "I don't want my son to get to know that I am a homosexual, and for him to be ashamed of me," he says. "I think that Allah will come to punish me."

Fazal, a 30-year-old mechanical engineer with an 18-year-old lover, prays that one day "I will see the light and stop this sin". His parents want to arrange for a wife for him, although he would rather choose one himself. "With time things change, and I might get used to a wife relationship," he says. He would like to move to Dubai, where he could live anonymously. "There I would not have to deal with the heartache of being despised and children calling me *msenge* on the street."

Others, such as Eric, believe that it is society rather than homosexual men who should change. But few would go as far as in Zimbabwe and Botswana or Europe and North America, where organisations of gay men have been established. The first attempt to form a gay club in Nairobi occurred in the 1960s, and Exotica was popular in the early 1970s until street fights erupted between women sex workers and gay men. Club 1900 emerged, but was hit by a government crackdown, with drugs cited as the reason. Today, there are places where men who have sex with men can meet, but information about them spreads clandestinely. Since homosexuality in Kenya is a criminal act, few men are willing to 'come out' – to admit their homosexuality openly and to demand a place for gay men in society.

Men, women and condoms

Some wives know of their husband's sexual and emotional relationships with other men. Amin, the primary school headmaster, for example, has an unspoken agreement with his wife of 26 years. She knows that he prefers men, and that he "bothered with her" only to have their three children. Karim in Mombasa has sexual relations with his wife on Wednesdays and Saturdays, but does not enjoy it; if she walked away from their marriage, he says, he would not bother to marry again. Of those wives who find out that their husbands are bisexual, some seek counselling, hoping that their husband will change. Those who are financially independent walk out.

The extent to which women are at risk of contracting HIV from their husbands' affairs is unclear. Often there is little sexual contact between them, although even one act of intercourse may transmit the virus if a condom is not used. A few men are careful to protect themselves and their wives by using condoms with their male partners. Others believe they are not at risk. Abdul, mentioned above, does not use condoms because "I am faithful to my partner and to my wife."

With no official information to guide them, few men who have sex with men use condoms on a regular basis. Some of the men interviewed said that they did not use condoms with their wives on the grounds that to do so would invite suspicion. Furthermore, they argued, there was no risk if they had only one male partner to whom they are faithful. (In fact, there is a risk if the partner is unfaithful or contracted HIV before the sexual relationship began.) Those who have multiple partners say they "try" to use condoms, but the word itself suggests they sometimes or often fail.

Of the men interviewed for this article, only Karim uses condoms all the time, although he finds them "cumbersome".. Others, such as Abdul and Fazal, consider that fidelity protects them. Odongo sees no need for protection, while Jared believes he is safe with young "untainted" boys. Amin occasionally uses condoms, believing that he cannot get HIV/AIDS if he goes out with "fresh" men. Kassim, 19, in Mombasa has just completed high school and would like to become a computer programmer. He admits that he has been promiscuous and that even though he is aware of AIDS he does not use a condom. "Why spoil the fun?" he asks, adding, "I hope that I won't get AIDS." Many of the men said they preferred sex without condoms. Others said regular condoms tore easily and that stronger condoms for homosexuals were not available in Kenya.

The threat of HIV

Kenya is severely affected by HIV/AIDS. An estimated 1.2 million Kenyans are believed to be HIV-positive and within the next three years up to 300,000 children will lose one or both parents to the disease. Child mortality is rising and adult life expectancy has fallen. The World Bank says that between two and four percent of the country's resources are spent on managing AIDS; some estimates say this might increase to 15 percent of the gross domestic product by the year 2000. Despite the threat there is a high level of denial and stigmatisation. Some 95 percent of Kenyans know about AIDS, yet only 20 to 30 percent have changed their sexual behaviour, according to Allan Ragi of the AIDS NGO Consortium.

While the authorities recognise the impact on the epidemic of male behaviour towards women, there is no official recognition of the role of men who have sex with men – who may either themselves contract HIV or pass the virus to their male or female partners. The fourth Sessional Paper on AIDS, adopted unanimously by Parliament in September 1997, acknowledges that "men's vulnerability is influenced by factors such as male ego", which drives them to risky sexual behaviour. Alcohol and substance abuse, labour migration and practices such as plural marriage are cited as additional factors that may lead to higher risk.. The closest the paper comes to admitting the existence of male-male sexual behaviour is the statement that "Groups such as beach boys, watchmen, soldiers, prisoners and truck drivers may usually establish casual relationships because circumstances separate them from their regular sexual partners for long periods. This makes them more vulnerable to HIV."

The Ministry of Health does not intend to allocate resources to HIV/AIDS interventions for men who have sex with men. The head of the Ministry's division of communicable diseases, Dr Maina Kahindo, considers that "taking into account other modes of transmission of HIV/AIDS, homosexuality is negligible, and should not take up our resources and time." He adds, "The only Kenyan men who engage in homosexuality are those who are in special circumstances which drive them to have sex with other men. Men having sex with a man occurs in schools, prisons and other institutions where the men have no access to the opposite sex. It is not really a sexual preference for Kenyan men. We have other, far more pressing areas which affect the majority of our people and therefore need urgent attention."

Dr Kahindo's comments are at odds with the evidence of the many men interviewed for this chapter. The government ignores the existence of male-male sexual behaviour, and there is no attempt to prevent HIV transmission even where the authorities recognise that sex between men occurs. Condom distribution in prisons or in the military has not been seriously proposed or discussed.

Growing awareness

While government recognition is yet to come, there is a slowly growing awareness among international and non-governmental organisations (NGOs) in Kenya that some men do have sex with other men. However, there is little agreement as to whether this behaviour should be accepted or changed, and programmes incorporating the specific needs of men who have sex with men are only just beginning.

Some church-based organisations offer medical, counselling and even financial support to men who are HIV positive and who have sex with men. MAP International, a Christian NGO that offers counselling on sexually transmitted diseases, says it welcomes all who seek help, including homosexuals. "The church has an obligation to these people," says Mike Wamae, a programme officer. He adds, "We think homosexuality is abnormal, but the mere fact that they are different does not mean that we would not become involved." However, he emphasises that assistance is given on the understanding that the men involved have the aim of stopping their "abnormal practices".

"We are dealing with human experiences and attitudes," says psychologist Protasia Gathendoh, who works at the Amani Counselling Centre, a Christian NGO in Nairobi. "We look at what makes an individual seek assistance, and we go from there. We try not to have a judgmental attitude." AMREF is currently evaluating HIV/AIDS cases in an effort to establish how people contracted the virus and then to develop more effective strategies for tackling the disease. According to the organisation's Dr Nduba, "Homosexuality is an area that needs to be looked into, but we tend to shy away from reality."

UNAIDS Resident Advisor George Tembo says his organisation has not yet targeted men who have sex with men. "It is a matter of priorities. There is no impact of AIDS campaigns yet on heterosexual behaviour to curb the spread of AIDS. Despite the campaigns, more and more Kenyans continue to be infected with HIV/AIDS. About 90 percent of AIDS in Kenya result from heterosexual activity. This is the area we are concentrating on." Tembo says that "homosexuals are not easily accessible. They will need to come out of the closet if they are to get any attention." In future, he notes, UNAIDS will try to offer support to homosexuals.

Whatever their attitudes, all representatives of organisations working on HIV/AIDS expressed interest in a study of the occurrence of homosexuality in the country. In addition to the lifestyles described in this article, it is clear that 'institutional homosexuality' – sexual activity between men in institutions such as boarding schools, the military and prisons – is worthy of research.

Meanwhile, public attitudes may be slowly changing. John Githongo, a columnist with the weekly *East African*, has argued for greater tolerance towards men who have sex with men. In a 1995 column he wrote: "The notion that the police can monitor and combat homosexuality is frightening. Kenyans as a whole are extremely heterosexual people, and we shouldn't get our knickers in a twist at the antics of a tiny minority behind closed doors" [12]. To outsiders this response may be patronising, but in Kenyan terms it is progress indeed.

IN A COUNTRY WHERE
NOBODY CARES

INTRODUCTION

Recreational drugs – substances which are eaten, drunk, inhaled or injected in order to alter physical sensations and mental attitudes – have been taken in every society since before recorded history. Coca leaf is chewed in the Andes, qat in the Horn of Africa; coffee is drunk in London, beer in Lusaka; marijuana cakes are eaten in Amsterdam, mescalin cactus in Mexico; crack cocaine is smoked in New York, tobacco in Beijing; heroin is injected in St Petersburg, a paste of pharmaceutical pills in São Paulo; sedatives are prescribed in Cairo and stimulants in Kingston.

Their impact varies. Some are relatively mild, others are more powerful and a few can cause serious physical damage. The legality also varies. Alcohol is banned in some countries and in recent years restrictions have begun to be placed on the use of tobacco. Opium and marijuana were freely available in the 19th century; for most of this century their use has been increasingly criminalised. Only very recently has the prohibition on marijuana been relaxed in some countries.

Legality is only one of a range of factors that determine the extent to which a drug is used. Often it is not difficult to obtain alcohol in countries where it is banned, while illegal drug use flourishes even in countries such as the United States, where hundreds of millions of dollars have been spent on the so-called 'war on drugs'. Perhaps the most powerful driving force behind drug use is the ability of producers and traders to make a profit – and the more addictive a drug, the more likely consumers will buy again and again. Social attitudes also play a major role. Cigarette smoking increases when it is seen as acceptable or desirable, while for many young men the initial attraction of injecting recreational drugs stems from the illegality of the practice.

Why men inject

Worldwide, between six and seven million people are believed to inject drugs regularly; 80 percent of them are men [1]. Injecting drug users are not a homogeneous group. Some inject on a daily basis for years, others irregularly or for a short period. Some maintain stable homes and careers while others lead chaotic lives, depending on crime or prostitution to pay for their habit. Those who have homes and are in control of their addiction are more likely to inject there, while the homeless or desperate must do so in the street or in the homes of dealers, where needles★ are frequently shared.

Researchers explain the preponderance of male drug injectors in several ways. According to one, "Men are more likely than women to partake in all forms of socially deviant behaviour, from illicit drug use to bank robberies. The only notable exception is sex work" [2]. Another comments: "Using [recreational] drugs is a selfish, inward-looking pursuit, aimed at artificial induction of a rewarding sensory state. It is at odds with the conventional nurturant role of women in society. They are expected to care for others and not exhibit sensual hedonism. Loss of control is regarded as particularly unattractive in women"[3]. Other explanations include men's greater economic resources.

★ As elsewhere in this book, the term 'needle' includes all parts of the manufactured or makeshift syringe where blood may mingle with the drug to be injected.

Drugs and HIV

Transmission of HIV is closely linked to the use of recreational drugs, injected or not. Drugs such as alcohol, used around the world, and 'crystal', currently common in the United States, lower inhibitions, making sexual encounters more likely and condom use less likely. Addiction also leads many women and men to resort to prostitution to earn the money to buy more drugs, and the desperation behind the act often prevents them from insisting on safer sex.

Injection of drugs, however, has a more direct impact on the course of the AIDS epidemic. Where users share equipment, the process of injecting almost always leaves a trace of an individual's blood in the needle or syringe. If that blood carries HIV, the chances that the virus will be transmitted to the next user(s), unless the equipment is thoroughly sterilised [4], is more than 1 in 200 [5]. Where the use of sterile syringes and needles is uncommon, HIV transmission can rise dramatically, as happened in Ho Chi Minh City, Vietnam, where infection rates among drug injectors leapt from one percent in 1992 to 39 percent in 1996 [6].

Because four times as many men as women inject drugs, men's drug-taking and sexual behaviour has a far greater impact on the HIV/AIDS epidemic. Women are more likely to restrict their injecting and sexual partners to the men with whom they are emotionally involved, while men are more likely to have sex with women who do not themselves inject [7]. Furthermore, an international survey in 1993 indicated that most men who inject never use condoms during sex [8].

Yet although rates of infection may be high within a group of drug users and their sexual partners, the virus may not extend far into the general population. This is partly because injectors and their partners, particularly if they are poor, are "a relatively immobile population that depends on a strong network of neighborhood residential and social ties to maintain contacts with … drug suppliers" [9]. The frequency of injections among this population makes it highly likely that many of them will contract HIV, while infrequent intercourse and sharing of needles with others reduces the likelihood that 'outsiders' will become infected. Nevertheless, this picture does not describe every drug injector and those who can afford to travel have undoubtedly played a part in the spread of virus within countries and across borders over the last 20 years.

Preventing transmission of HIV

There are two broad approaches to the prevention of HIV among injecting drug users. One is to enforce strong policing strategies to stop users from acquiring the drug in question and the equipment with which to inject it; this can be seen in its most extreme form in countries where conviction for certain drug-related offences results in the death penalty. The other approach, known as 'harm reduction', is to educate users to sterilise their equipment and to provide sterile equipment through needle-exchange – the distribution of syringes or the exchange of new syringes for old. These approaches frequently lead to animated debate like that surrounding condom use. Opponents of the supply of sterile needles argue that it stimulates demand and encourages dangerous and illegal behaviour, while those in favour argue that since the 'war on drugs' has not been won [10], the best policy is to reduce the potential harm from injecting.

Slowly, however, increasing political support is being given to needle exchange, as a result of increasing evidence that it works. A recent study of 81 cities worldwide indicated that HIV infection among drug injectors increased by an average of 5.9 percent in cities without needle exchange programmes, and declined 5.8 percent in cities with programmes [11].

Needle exchange is only part of the solution. Achieving the goal of ensuring that injectors' equipment is always sterile may be hampered by the attitudes of users themselves. The need to inject may be so overwhelming that the user pays no attention to the state of the equipment, and for a few users the ritual of sharing equipment is an important part of the experience, irrespective of the risks of infection. Strategies to overcome this obstacle include introducing sterilisation as part of the ritual and suggesting that those who know or suspect that they are HIV-positive inject last, to avoid passing the virus to others.

Changing times in Russia

Patterns of drug use can change rapidly within a short period, and thousands who do not inject one year may begin to do so the next, with disastrous results for themselves, their partners and the communities in which they live. This was the case in Thailand when the widespread habit of smoking opium derivatives was overtaken by the fashion of injecting the drug; within a year HIV infection among drug users in Bangkok rose from one percent to over 30 percent [12].

For many years alcohol was the most widely abused substance in Russia, but the situation changed radically with the social and economic changes following the collapse of the Soviet Union. "Two or three years ago we had one drug user for every 10 kids with a drinking problem," says Pyotr Belaskov, a doctor in a narcotics treatment centre in Moscow. "Now it's the other way round." The following report examines the lives of some of those who have been physically or psychologically addicted to drugs, and the steps being taken to reduce the risk of HIV transmission among those who inject.

MEN, INJECTED DRUGS AND HIV/AIDS IN RUSSIA

by Kester Kenn Klomegah

Kaliningrad, a depressed Baltic port of one million people. A filthy basement near the train station, filled with a suffocating mix of iodine vapour, petrol fumes and cigarette smoke. Dima and Sergey, both in their early twenties, are sprawled on a bench. A syringe shakes in Dima's hand as he injects another dose of an opaque liquid into his vein. Dima passes the blood-stained needle to Sergey, whose eyes are focused on the small vial. As the needle enters his arm, three more men and a woman arrive to inject drugs in their turn. "Let's have a good time," Dima screams.

In the last decade Kaliningrad has become the entry point for much of Russia's imported heroin and cocaine. This basement, however, is far removed from the world of smuggling and criminal gangs. Dima and his friends are injecting a locally produced opiate, the cost dramatically less than imported narcotics and the risk of detection minimal. On other occasions they might inject cocaine or amphetamines ground into a paste, the cheapest alternative. While heroin costs US$100 per gram, a dozen pills of relanium, a sedative, can be bought for only US$7. None of those present know if they are HIV-positive. They probably are, but in their euphoric state none of them care.

A tenfold increase

Russian society continues to reverberate from the impact of the collapse of the Soviet Union in 1991. Radical social and economic change has led to widespread unemployment, poverty and a relaxation of social and legal taboos. This, coupled with an influx of illegal drugs, has led to a rapid rise in the number of injecting drug users, a trend shadowed by a steep increase in the number of Russians who have contracted HIV.

Vladimir Yegorov, a drugs expert at the Ministry of Health, estimates there are between 500,000 and 700,000 injecting drug addicts nationwide, 10 times more than the 1995 estimate of 64,000 addicts and over 20 times higher than in 1990. Yegorov believes that another five million people inject drugs irregularly. Many users begin injecting in their mid-teens, a psychologically vulnerable age. In Kaliningrad in 1996, for example, the number of registered drug users under 19 increased by 36 percent; one survey indicates that a majority of 16-17 year olds in the city have tried the locally produced opiate at least once [13].

As the number of addicts rises, so does the number of people living with HIV. Only three of the 1,542 Russians known to be HIV-positive in 1995 had contracted the virus through drug injection; by November 1997 the Health Ministry had been notified of 4,500 cases of HIV infection, 62 percent of whom were drug users. In a parallel epidemic, 80 percent of drug users tested positive for hepatitis B [14].

The official figures are believed to be a fraction of the real total. An estimated one million people will be living with the virus in 2000 [15], the vast majority of whom will have contracted HIV through drug injection or through sexual intercourse with an HIV-positive drug user. Meanwhile the epidemic, currently worst in western cities with strong international links such as St Petersburg and Moscow, has already begun to spread, with increasing numbers of cases in cities in Siberia and the east.

Men at risk

Most drug users – and therefore most people known to be HIV-positive – are men, and most are young. Nikolai Nedzelsky, president of the non-governmental organisation IMENA, has several theories to explain why men are more likely to inject drugs and to be reported as contracting HIV. "In our Russian family, women are more dependent on men. A man allows himself to do whatever he wants in the family, but a woman can't afford this." This freedom applies both to drug injection and sexual intercourse. Because they expect to contract infections, Nedzelsky argues, men are more likely to attend STD clinics, which also leads to detection of more cases of sexual transmission of HIV among men than among women.

Nedzelsky also points out that while young women stay with their parents, many young men who inject drugs live with other users. When their apartments are raided by the police, those arrested are identified as addicts and made to undergo an HIV test. Both facts are reported to the Health Ministry.

This apparent bias aside, Nedzelsky and other experts believe that men do in fact comprise the majority of drug users and people with HIV. Closer examination of the circumstances that lead men to inject and to contract the virus suggests that this will remain the situation in Russia for the foreseeable future.

"A form of art"

Ask young men why they take drugs and the answers are unclear. Dima in Kaliningrad prefers drugs to alcohol because they are "more spiritual". Kostya, a 20-year-old in a dirt-stained black leather jacket, responds: "We're in a country where nobody cares about anything. Who cares if I say I'm on drugs? It's my decision and up to me to choose the way I want to live." Vadim, 21, has a similarly casual attitude: "Why do I take drugs? I don't know. Maybe to get high, to visit another planet," while Anton, who does not give his age, says: "Personally, I see drug use as a form of art rather than a science."

Yevgeny Tolkachev, deputy director of Moscow Narcotics Hospital No 17, offers another analysis: "Most drug users we have dealt with are targets in three senses even before they try any drugs: their social circumstances are unstable, they are psychologically inclined to respond to the attraction of drugs and their metabolism is particularly disposed towards the physical effects."

The greatest influence, however, must be the social and economic changes of the 1990s. Yuri Buida, a sociologist with the literary journal *Znamya*, sees the rise in the use of drugs as "evidence of the democratisation and liberalisation of a society living through a severe crisis of traditional values". Nikolai Nedzelsky says, "All the values that we used to have in this country have been destroyed. When I was at school I knew that I would be able to go to an institute, graduate from it, find an interesting job, build a certain career. Today youngsters do not know what they are living for."

Nedzelsky points out that drugs are everywhere. "The 'narcotisation' of society is obvious all around you. Wherever you go – nightclubs, discos and just in the street – you always run across drug users, drug sellers and so on." The situation has got so bad that "here in Russia even old women go in for drug selling. In the marketplace they stand with a knapsack and sell ready-made portions in syringes, and no one knows who used this disposable syringe before."

"It's not enough to have one's own syringe"

Given the circumstances in which most drug injection occurs, it is not surprising that it has swiftly led to HIV transmission. Oleg, a 24-year-old who has given up drugs after years of addiction, explains: "It's not enough just to have one's own syringe to protect oneself. One can get infected from a common spoon if the solution itself is infected. If we talk about *vint* [a commonly injected metamphetamine-based drug], the 'cook' who makes it can use an infected syringe – infected with hepatitis or anything else. Everyone who injects it will get infected. Or say if I take heroin, it is cooked in a spoon. If anyone takes his share first with an infected syringe and I take mine after him, even with a newly opened syringe – that'll be it, I'll get infected, no matter what kind of syringe I use."

Awareness of AIDS has increased sharply in recent years but it seldom has an impact on users' behaviour. As Oleg says, "If I sit with a fellow user and we use the same syringe, the first thing I'd think about would be how fast to inject it. Afterwards I might think about whether he is ill or not." But, he emphasises, he will think about it only when it is too late to prevent possible infection.

"Shooting up and having sex"

It is difficult to confirm the extent to which HIV among drug users is passed to their sexual partners. Anton, a young man in his early twenties, says that three times a day his first priority is to inject drugs. Then he looks for girls. "The only things on my mind are shooting up and having sex." The previous week, he claims, he had sex with four different women. The drug Anton and his friend Dmitri use is a crude opiate mixed with an antihistamine. Sometimes one or more women injects with them and both men have sex with them. It is not difficult, he claims, to find women who offer sex in exchange for drugs.

Sasha, 24, cannot count the number of women drug users with whom he has had sex. "When it's happening, we can't control ourselves," he says. "I don't keep track of how often or with whom." Dr Alexander Dreyzin, deputy director of the Narcotics Hospital in Kaliningrad, suggests that group sex is an integral aspect of drug taking. "It's part of the culture. It may be sex between men or men sharing one or more female partners."

Anton and Sasha may be exaggerating and Dreyzin's information may be inaccurate, but Russians in general have active sex lives. A survey by condom manufacturers London International Group suggests that out of 15 countries, Russia is the third most sexually active [16]. Condoms are widely available but the survey ranked Russia 12th in the frequency of condom use, and a study conducted by the Health Ministry in the early 1990s found that only 10 percent of the population use them on a regular basis. According to the Ministry, three quarters of teenagers are unaware that condoms should not be used more than once, and many do not understand how sexual diseases are transmitted.

As a result sexually transmitted infections (STIs) are spreading rapidly, with over 150,000 reported cases in Moscow alone in 1996. Nationwide, 400,000 Russians were estimated to have syphilis in 1997, a 60-fold increase in eight years [17]. Despite these figures most Russians believe that HIV and other STIs are common only among foreigners and national minorities. "Young people do not understand HIV very well and some teenagers even wonder whether AIDS is really so dangerous," says Dr Alexandre Fuzeau, a French specialist in the disease working in Moscow.

Four more years

Once addicted, most injectors find themselves on a road towards death that offers few opportunities for escape. Vladimir Yegorov of the Health Ministry claims the average lifespan for those who inject is no more than 40. Nikolai Nedzelsky of

IMENA is more pessimistic, quoting research that indicates that addicts live an average of only four years after they first inject. (Information from New York City suggests that on average addicts there live for 20 years [18].) Death comes, Zedzelsky says, from an overdose, an accident caused by drug use or hepatitis B; those who survive find they have lost many of their friends.

AIDS compounds the prognosis, and while addicts know that it is difficult but not impossible to stop injecting, HIV appears to extinguish the last vestige of hope. "Why would I bother with an AIDS test?" 29-year-old Yura asks. "Even if I have it, so what? The effect will be exactly the same either way. Death" [19].

Yevgeny Voronin, head of the AIDS Centre for Russia in St Petersburg, illustrates the impact of AIDS on the youngest, most vulnerable users: "A kid of 17 or 18 gets told he's HIV-positive and can't be treated. Naturally, when he gets this scary diagnosis, he realises there is absolutely nothing left for him to be scared of. He disappears." This means, Voronin adds, that he does not care whether he uses clean needles. "The situation will only get worse until we start offering drug addicts something in return" [20].

The cost of treatment

So far the authorities appear unable to reduce either the spread of HIV or the numbers who take up the needle. Vladimir Yegorov, the leading narcotics expert in the Health Ministry, admits that the state is failing to rehabilitate drug users. Hospital withdrawal programmes appear to have little impact. Yevgeny Tolkachev of Moscow Narcotics Hospital No 17 says, "If we got these kids in the early stages, we could do something. But we get them only when their problem has become a full-grown addiction, so they stay in hospital for little more than a quick breather from their habit."

Yegorov claims that the average drug user does not seek

medical aid for addiction until five to seven years after first taking drugs, by which time a full rehabilitation programme is necessary. Drug users' contacts with other people have become limited, their social ties have broken up and these and other changes in lifestyle cannot be altered in a few days with pills. "Rehabilitation centres are necessary to help drug users change their lifestyles and moral values and, most importantly, learn some vocation that would help them to settle in life." However, this level of treatment costs US$200 per patient per day, a sum far beyond the means of Russia's failing health service. The situation is even more critical in the provinces, which have fewer resources than are available in the capital and in the more developed cities in the west of the country.

Yegorov recognises that users require more than medical help, but his attitude does not appear to be shared by most of the help providers. Nikolai Nedzelsky tells the story of a drug user with tissue decay who sought medical assistance. "He said he was treated like an outcast and they did surgical operations without any anaesthetic, saying, 'Well, you're a drug user, you've already got your portion of anaesthetic.'" Oleg, quoted above, spent 28 days in Hospital 17. "You'd get haloperidol injections and for two days you'd lie down in a horrible state. When relief comes, convulsions start. Then they wrote a diagnosis, 'drug addiction', and I was registered. Doctors just mock you. No moral support. Most of the addicts go to hospitals just to survive the 'cold turkey' [withdrawal] period if they don't have money for methadone. Then they go back out and get high again."

"The philosophy of our masters seems to be that the average drug addict dies within four or five years anyway, so what's the point of treating him for AIDS when there are 'normal' people needing treatment. They say the US$10,000 a year treatment cost is too high, although no one says it's too expensive to pay US$70,000 a year for kidney dialysis," says Yevgeny Voronin [21].

The wrong approach

Nikolai Nedzelsky claims that the health authorities have the wrong approach to drug use. "The official structures try to prohibit the use of drugs. And anti-drug propaganda is much, much weaker than the promotion of drugs. I can understand a 15-year-old when he hears from the TV, 'Don't use drugs, it's bad for you,' and when he hears a friend saying that he tried it and it's such bliss: definitely his friend's words will impress him more. Therefore it's necessary to change state policy as a whole. Rather than simply frightening people, as they love to do in this country, give them true information about what drugs are and how to protect yourself."

With almost no social or medical support, drug users must rely on their own will to break free of addiction. In Nedzelsky's words: "The more a man uses drugs, the more he becomes aware that on the one hand it could be fatal and on the other he is tired of the habit because there's no money, everything he had is ruined. Some people feel that drugs are affecting their brains, and gradually they give them up. The people I know who gave up didn't go to official medical establishments, because in most cases the treatment is discriminatory and ineffective. It tries to help cope with the physical addiction but not the psychological one."

Nedzelsky warns that although parents often try to help sons or daughters withdraw from drugs, "there's a certain danger" if a child is accepted for treatment. "There are experienced addicts there and in fact he would learn the whole system of drug distribution, how to buy them, how to sell them, how he can get the purest drug etc." Oleg's experience in Narcotics Hospital 17 confirms this: "I got nothing but new acquaintances and information on new places where I could buy drugs and find new dealers."

New steps

The national authorities appear to have taken no action to confront the rapidly worsening situation. In 1997 the government failed to allocate the negligible sum of US$46,000 budgeted for the AIDS Prevention and Treatment Centre's programme. Meanwhile, international and non-governmental efforts to limit the spread of HIV among drug users have only recently begun and are inadequate for the task.

Despite lack of a tradition of outreach programmes and initial fears that the social workers and the drug users they advise would be subject to arrest, such a programme has been launched in St Petersburg by the Return Foundation. This includes a special bus offering advice on drug use, medical help and needle exchanges. The bus has received an enormous response, suggesting there is a strong demand for information and help if the approach is right. A similar programme has begun in the city of Yaroslavl.

The paucity of services available is evident in the fact that drug users across the country who test positive for HIV are recommended by their home authorities to go to the Return Foundation's bus. "You get HIV-positive people coming from all over Russia to St Petersburg, including addicts who then go to the market in town and shoot up with our local kids. As soon as an HIV-positive person is sent to our city, the risk here grows. It's illogical," says Grigory Latyshev, the Foundation coordinator [22].

International experience has shown that the political leaders who could take decisive action to prevent HIV from gaining more than a foothold almost never act until it is too late. Russia looks like being no exception. If current trends continue (as they are almost certain to do) this country, which once offered global leadership, may begin the new century crippled by the overwhelming social and economic costs of one of the world's worst AIDS epidemics.

HELL ON EARTH

INTRODUCTION

In every society groups of people such as refugees and other immigrants, ethnic minorities and prisoners confront daily hardships unknown to the majority of the population. The very existence of these groups is often ignored or forgotten by the majority. Their hardships often include greater vulnerability to HIV.

In many countries the number of prisoners is high: Russia's 1.35 million prisoners in 1996 [1] represented about one adult in 50. The numbers are often growing, too: the 1.6 million men and women incarcerated in the United States in 1995 (more than one in 100 adults) represent a doubling since 1985 [2]. The fact that the vast majority of prisoners are men reflects men's tendency to take risks and transgress society's norms more than women.

The primary purpose of prison is to punish. Many argue that prison should also reform, so that when inmates return to the outside world they do not break the law again. Frequently, however, little attempt is made to reform, and housing young prisoners with older, experienced offenders creates schools of crime whose graduates are even more likely to offend. In addition, conditions in many prisons are so poor that the punishment inmates receive is often far in excess of their offence. Overcrowding leads to unsanitary conditions, disease and violent tension; for some inmates, contracting infection with HIV is an additional, unexpected sentence. Tuberculosis, which thrives where there is HIV, is another hazard.

HIV in prison

Many prisoners of both sexes have a history of injecting drugs, which often leads to a higher HIV prevalence in prisons than in the population at large. Needles* are scarce, illegal and difficult to hide; often home-made from such items as ballpoint pens, they are almost always shared. In male prisons HIV is also transmitted through sexual activity [3]; condoms are rarely available and the risk of transmission is heightened if violent intercourse or lack of lubrication leads to bleeding. Surveys in Australia, Canada, England and Zambia suggest six to 12 percent of men in prison have sex — "figures which are probably low because of denial and under-reporting" [4]. Other surveys indicate that more than half of Nigerian prisoners have "at least one current sexual partner" [5], and studies quoted in this chapter report that over 70 percent of men in prison in Brazil and Costa Rica are sexually active.

Sex in prisons may be consensual or coerced. The extent to which rape of male prisoners occurs in any country is uncertain. Certainly, Brazil is not an exception. One specialist from the International Committee of the Red Cross describes what may be typical situations in Russia — "Unspeakable forms of what can only be described as sexual depravity are inflicted on [some] prisoners, for reasons of sexual gratification and sheer perversity" — and in the United States, where "the sexual abuse of male prisoners by other male prisoners is more than just a serious problem" [6].

Against such a background it is not surprising that HIV prevalence in prisons is usually high, nor that it is a significant factor in prison mortality. In France inmates are 10 times more likely to be HIV-positive than the general population; in the United States the figure is six times [7]. In 1992 a full 24 percent of all deaths in US state prisons were due to AIDS [8]. According to the report below, AIDS is responsible for well over half the mortality in Brazilian prisons. Whether the virus was contracted

*   As elsewhere in this book, 'needle' refers to any and all parts of the equipment used to inject drugs.

before or during imprisonment is irrelevant; for every inmate with HIV, conditions in jail hasten the development of symptoms, and the lack of appropriate treatment and drugs increases the likelihood of early death.

Prison staff and society at large are also put at risk. Staff may contract HIV through sexual intercourse with the prisoners, as punishment or in exchange for rewards, and through injuries from contact with needles during searches of prisoners' property. A greater risk is faced by the sexual and drug-injecting partners of prisoners, during conjugal visits or on their release from jail. If only one percent of Brazilian inmates contract HIV while in jail, that figure still represents 250 men who return home each year and risk passing the newly acquired infection to other men and women. The actual figure is likely to be much higher.

Condoms, needles and violence

HIV/AIDS prevention workers have long argued that condoms and sterile needles should be distributed to inmates, but many prison authorities continue to resist this policy [9]. The grounds for resistance are similar to other situations in which condom and needle distribution are proposed: that to do so condones or encourages illegal behaviour. But the scale of drug injection and sex in some prisons suggests there is little scope for further encouragement of such behaviour. In any case, even if — and there is no evidence to prove this is the case — some individuals begin injecting or sexual activity as a result of condom and needle distribution, it is surely a small price to pay for the number of lives that will be saved. It is likely, however, that condoms will make an impact only when the underlying question of sexual violence in prisons is resolved [10].

Mário Scheffer and Marcelo Marthe describe a number of projects intended to reduce HIV transmission in prison. Prisoners also need to develop the personal and social skills to build self-respect and lifestyles that will help them avoid returning to prison after their release. This is the focus of a number of projects in Central America based on a model developed by the non-

governmental organisation ILPES in San José, Costa Rica. The projects begin by helping prisoners understand and prevent HIV transmission, and move into areas such as the understanding and prevention of violence in prison and the development of inmates' artisanal skills.

An earlier version of this report, commissioned by Panos, was published in Brazil in early 1998, leading to a promise by the authorities that action would be taken to reduce HIV transmission among inmates. Some of the details of this article may therefore be out of date by the time the book appears. Whether or not conditions do change in Brazil, many countries will see their own experiences reflected here.

MEN IN PRISON IN BRAZIL

by Mário Scheffer & Marcelo Marthe

In August 1996 in Carandiru prison, São Paulo state, detainee Antonio Carlos Rosa claimed to have invented a medicine capable of curing a long list of illnesses, including AIDS. Mixing dirty water and disinfectant, Rosa prepared the mixture as instructed by God in a vision. He distributed the remedy to 110 volunteers, then revealed the results to the press. It was only then that the prison authorities learned of the experiment. Luckily, the so-called "pathological laxative" caused no harm other than diarrhoea. Rosa was sent to an asylum for the insane and shortly afterwards his case was filed and forgotten.

This macabre story, set in the largest prison in Latin America (with 6,000 inmates), gives an insight into the extent of the neglect suffered by Brazilian prisoners. The crazy experiment masked a cruel fact: for prisoners, lack of health care has passed the limits of desperation.

Brazil has about 250 prisons. A similar number of police stations act as improvised jails. Federal statistics state that

114,000 men, 5,000 women and 29,000 others (sex not notified) are incarcerated out of a population of 160 million. The prison population is predominantly under 30 years old, illiterate or semi-literate, and before arrest unemployed or living below the poverty line. In police cells up to 30 or 40 people — known as bat-men, because they hang in rows of hammocks from the walls and ceiling — are frequently stacked into cubicles of 20 square metres; inmates are locked in 24 hours a day, have little or no access to natural light, no leisure or work activities, appalling food and no medical attention. Prisons are less overcrowded and have facilities such as workshops and leisure space where games of soccer may be played.

Whether in prison or a police cell, however, inmates with AIDS, tuberculosis, hepatitis, sexually transmitted diseases (STDs) or any other illness find themselves on the bottom rung of a social ladder. Excluded by a system in which poverty and lack of education frequently leads to crime, these men and women have no access to even the minimum rights guaranteed by law. Many end up staying in jail much longer than their sentence, and are at risk of contracting HIV through shared syringes or sex without condoms. As a result, according to Ricardo Marins, an epidemiologist with the University of Campinas, AIDS has become the principal cause of death in these outposts of hell, killing more even than violence and tuberculosis.

HIV in prisons

By early 1998 it was estimated that 500,000 Brazilians (0.6 percent of the adult population) were living with HIV. In Carandiru prison, 17.3 percent of detainees had the virus; in Sorocaba prison in São Paulo state, the rate was 12.5 percent. Overall, the Health Ministry believes that about 22,000 prisoners (15 percent of the total) are HIV-positive. One expert, Pedro Chequer, coordinator of the Ministry of

A Mediaeval Dungeon

"I learnt I had AIDS four years ago, when I was taken to the prison hospital with pneumonia. I didn't know the reason for all the tests they gave me. One afternoon the doctor, who had not appeared for several days, came and told me, 'You're going to die, because you have AIDS.' It was the worst moment of my life." The testimony of 28-year-old João da Silva, serving 14 years in Porto Alegre Central Prison for drug dealing, reveals the lack of ethics with which the majority of health professionals treat prisoners with HIV.

In Porto Alegre just three doctors, two nurses and 12 assistant nurses are responsible for the care of 3,000 prisoners. Of the 25 deaths registered in the prison in 1997, 21 were from AIDS. "Here we have to beg to be seen to," says one prisoner. "If you have AIDS you are taken to the prison hospital only when you are about to die." The AIDS block in Carandiru has 65 beds and receives patients from various prisons. In June 1997, 33 prisoners were interned there, 15 deaths were recorded and seven prisoners in the terminal stages of the disease were released. During one inspection by the Medical Council, the organisation responsible for upholding medical ethics, none of the 10 doctors who work at the prison was present. Receiving little more than US$500 for 20 hours' work, and with no medicines, gauze, sutures or anaesthetics, most doctors put in only two hours of work a week. With no police escorts to supervise transfers and with hospitals refusing to receive prisoners because of alleged lack of security, there is no treatment outside prison.

A report compiled by members of the Brazilian Congress in 1997 revealed that prisoners who could hardly move treated themselves by applying sugar and coffee to their wounds. Those who needed intravenous drips improvised with plastic straws. In the 18 months since he had entered prison, Paulo João de Souza had lived with a femur fracture that had not been operated on. One inmate had been shot in prison but the bullet had not been removed; he lay paralysed in the foetal position, with a serious urethral infection for which he had no antibiotics. Another prisoner, with advanced AIDS, was in agony, watched over by a companion in a wheelchair.

"The state meets neither the minimum United Nations recommendations nor our own country's laws," the parliamentarians' document concluded. After one visit a representative of the Order of Brazilian Lawyers commented: "What we saw was a mediaeval dungeon. There was no air to breathe. Human beings were rotting slowly in the humidity ... incomprehensible and unacceptable horror ... practice of slow extermination."

Not every prison hospital is so bad. The 28-bed Penitentiary Hospital in Niterói in Rio de Janeiro state is considered a model of good treatment. Doctors are always present (salary: US$1,120 for 20 hours), as well as nurses, a psychologist and a social worker. Basic materials, diagnostic tests and a range of anti-HIV drugs are available. However, if the patient's health improves he is returned to prison, where treatment may cease. According to Edison José Biondi, superintendent of the prison health system, "We give antiviral drugs to the prisoners, but many hand them on to their families and sell them outside the prison." ∎

Health's National STD/AIDS Programme, comments, "In fact, we don't know the real scale of the problem. The number of prisoners with HIV could be more than we imagine."

According to Paulo Junqueira, who oversees AIDS and prison policy in the Health Ministry, "It's very difficult to determine whether prisoners contract [HIV] more easily inside or outside prison. Outside, many inject drugs and have many sexual partners. But certainly the precarious conditions inside prison make prisoners very vulnerable to the epidemic." Specialists agree that injectable drugs are a more important risk factor than sex in disseminating HIV in prison. This is partly based on the assumption that if one in five of all Brazilians diagnosed with AIDS contracted the virus through injecting drugs, the rate must be much higher in prisons, where 28 percent of all prisoners are sentenced for drug-related crimes. Junqueira refines the picture: "There are no statistics on the number of prisoners who take drugs or have sex in prison. Every prison is different, and the situation in each depends on the local culture and incidence [of drug taking]. In Rio de Janeiro and the north and north-east regions, the incidence of drug taking is relatively low and most cases of HIV transmission will be sexual. In the south and São Paulo, most prisoners contract the virus through contaminated needles."

Most of the 115 prisoners with HIV interviewed by Ricardo Marins in Sorocaba admitted they had sexual relations in prison, almost always without the use of a condom. Half reported a sexually transmitted disease in the last five years, 20 percent injected cocaine and all had clinical complications caused by HIV, particularly pneumonia and tuberculosis. Preliminary research suggests that the survival rate for prisoners with the virus is much lower than for people with HIV who are not behind bars.

A valuable commodity

The most common drug in prison is marijuana. "The police themselves bring it in. More than once I saw a delivery of 10 or 15 kilos of marijuana," says Cláudio Badé dos Santos, who has seen the inside of half a dozen prisons and police cells. "The drug is always a gift, usually from an imprisoned drug baron. With so much dope, a guy can live comfortably, with various perks, and be feared by the other prisoners." After marijuana, Santos says, crack cocaine is the most common drug. "You mix it with bicarbonate of soda and water and smoke it in a makeshift pipe." It has an immediate effect, powerful but short-lived. A common, economical method of taking crack is to sprinkle a few pieces in a marijuana cigarette, which results in the popular 'mix'.

Drugs are almost always taken in a group. Up to 15 prisoners get together in a cell, taking turns to watch for the guards. "There is a camaraderie when you share the joint. Anyone who wants to do it on his own, or not with the gang of the man who supplied it, has to pay with packets of cigarettes or favours," says Santos. The scarcity of cocaine means that many prisoners prefer to inject rather than inhale it, using syringes and needles obtained from the refuse bins in the prison pharmacy.

"A syringe lasts a very long time," notes Santos. "A harpoon [syringe] is a valuable commodity, which ends up being used 20 to 25 times," according to João da Silva, from Porto Alegre. Santos says that syringes are washed out with water and passed from prisoner to prisoner. "If you can heat the water, fine. But it's usually cold water." His words are confirmed by research with 180 drug users in Porto Alegre Central Prison, which revealed that most did not clean syringes well enough to prevent transmission of HIV.

The imprisoned libido

There are two kinds of sex in Brazilian prisons: conjugal visits carried out with the approval of the authorities, and sex between prisoners.

Conjugal visits, during which a male prisoner can have sex with a female companion from outside, are treated as a privilege. Permission for such visits often depends on the goodwill of a guard. Usually the couple must provide proof they are married. Otherwise the guard must be bribed. In a few prisons, according to one authority, girlfriends and even the partners of homosexual prisoners are allowed in for private visits.

Until recently, conjugal visits in the São Paulo prison system were allowed only to those with a negative HIV test, on the grounds that this protected the prisoner's family. Similarly, until 1995 conjugal visits in Rio de Janeiro state were subject to a stipulation that both prisoner and visitor must have health certificates with evidence of a negative HIV test.

Conjugal visits are almost always consummated in the corner of a cell or courtyard, with the couple standing and covered by a sheet while other prisoners keep guard. "It's common for some prisoners to offer their wife or girlfriend to other prisoners to pay a debt or to get something in exchange, like money, drugs or other favours," says Victor, a prisoner on temporary parole. "I once saw a man offering his daughter to the boss of a cell."

Conjugal visits are not allowed in the police cells, but the ban can be overcome. "I was in a cell which was emptied to allow prisoners to meet their girlfriends," says Cláudio Santos. "You had to pay five reales (US$4.50) for the right to have sex. It couldn't take longer than 10 minutes, because there were a lot of prisoners. More than one couple did it at the same time, separated by only a sheet." The money collected was divided among the guards and the 'trusties' (prisoners with a record of good behaviour who assist the guards). "They even allowed prostitutes in for those prisoners who didn't have a girlfriend but who could pay."

Every year approximately 25,000 detainees regain their freedom, of whom 3,500 are likely to be HIV-positive. Many will have contracted the virus in prison. Most, according to Ricardo Marins's research, return to wives or girlfriends; those who are newly HIV-positive risk transmitting the virus to their partners and future children.

"Don't worry, someone will buy you"

Sex between prisoners is forbidden and, when detected, subject to severe punishment, such as solitary confinement and a diet of bread and water. It can be between men and women: during the seven months in which she was held in a mixed prison in Altamira, in the far north of Brazil, one woman prisoner was systematically raped by the 35 other prisoners in her cell. But it is more usually between two or more men, and anecdotal evidence suggests that the practice is widespread.

Informers, rapists and others accused of sexual crimes, particularly child abusers, rarely escape rape by other inmates. Some are victims only once; others are attacked systematically. "It happens more often in police cells than in the large prisons," says Santos. "When guys get as far as prison, the crime they committed has usually been forgotten, or they have been 'paid back' enough for it to be ignored."

Rape is also the punishment for those who cause trouble, steal or accumulate debts to pay for drugs. The bodies of transvestites [11] and effeminate men become a currency worth trading. One transsexual, who wished to remain anonymous, spent eight months in Carandiru. "Soon after I got there, the bosses began to negotiate. Are you a transvestite? Effeminate queer? Don't worry, someone will buy you." The individual concerned receives a sum of money and sleeps besides his 'owner', who has sex with him on demand. There is no choice. Sometimes his 'lover' rents him to other inmates.

High turnover and overcrowding in police cells allows transvestites and effeminate men the alternative of prostitution. Valerie, from São Paulo, spent eight months behind bars. "I didn't have an 'owner' but I sold myself. I had sex for five reales or for drugs, packets of cigarettes or food, which my clients got from their visitors. I already had HIV, but I didn't use a condom, because there were none available."

Prison guards may be involved in such transactions. And while transvestites and openly homosexual men may be exploited in prison, there are situations in which the opposite is true. Guards may offer sex in exchange for favours, as when a transsexual asks to change cells. Sometimes the guard is the penetrator; sometimes he asks a prisoner to 'screw' him in exchange for drugs or other privileges.

Topmen, Possums and Chickens

From our in-depth interviews [in 1990 in a Costa Rican prison], it became evident that 70 to 90 percent of inmates have sexual relationships. Those interviewed reported an average of 51 sexual partners in the previous six months. One reported sex with 365 partners. Prison officials also report high percentages. We can identify various types of homosexual relationships in prison:

1. The *cachero* (topman) and the transvestite: the *cachero* is the masculine man who is supposedly the anal penetrator in a homosexual relationship.
2. The older man and the *cabrito* (chicken): the cabrito is a young, often beardless, adolescent. The older man provides money and protection; the sexual practice varies.
3. Two closet homosexuals [12] (called *zorras* — possums — in Costa Rica): this relationship is based more on mutual reciprocity than on power.

Although these are steady relationships involving intercourse, the partners may have occasional contact with other prisoners. Broadly speaking, men can be divided into those who are insertive and those who are receptive, and homosexual relations are accepted only between these two groups. It is not accepted (though it sometimes happens) for two masculine or two effeminate men to get together.

Nevertheless, it is not sexual practice that determines who is a *cachero* in jail, but power as a gang leader or as a dangerous and violent man. While the *cachero* can experiment sexually and be anally penetrated by a transvestite or a youth, he is still a *cachero* with the capacity to kill. No one dares question his masculinity as a result of these variations in his sexual behaviour. He is not defined as a homosexual. A very young *cachero* is not respected by older men and may be raped to demonstrate that he should not mess with transvestites or other effeminate men.

Jacobo Schifter, Johnny Madrigal, Peter Aggleton [13]

Preventing transmission

Nationwide, about 200 NGOs have developed HIV/AIDS prevention projects targeted at segments of the population considered to be at risk. Very few, however, are for prisoners, since the 29 state governments primarily responsible for prison conditions are often reluctant to admit the existence of activities which transmit HIV. Furthermore, police cells are the responsibility of the municipalities. "There are various people that have to be dealt with when developing a prevention programme for detainees. That is without taking into account petty officials, such as directors, long-term guards who have accumulated power in prison, and leaders of organised crime who have been imprisoned and who have authority in some prisons. There are always difficult negotiations before any project begins," says Paulo Junqueira of the Ministry of Health.

Prisons seldom allow the distribution and exchange of syringes. On one occasion a specialist who had given a lecture about the dangers of drugs distributed four syringes in Porto Alegre Central Prison, a one-off experiment with potentially dangerous consequences. Some medical staff have tried to convince prison directors to stock cleaning liquids containing hypochloride solution, in the hope that the product might also be used for needle hygiene. The solution may not eliminate HIV but it is more efficient than water, and such an approach may be the only way of reducing the impact of shared needles in the foreseeable future.

Rio de Janeiro state has the only prevention programme relating to conjugal visits. Project Conjugal Visit stipulates that the selected detainees and their sexual partners must attend lectures on topics such as family planning, contraception and sexually transmitted diseases. In addition, an educational video is shown and booklets and condoms distributed. Every prison in the state has a social worker and psychologist to monitor the programme.

Since mid-1997 the state government of São Paulo has authorised the distribution of 100,000 condoms a month in its prisons. Officially they are for use during conjugal visits, but given that the programme aims to reach most of the 36,000 prisoners in the state system, the authorities are implicitly acknowledging other situations in which the condoms might be used. However, poor relations between the body responsible for health in prisons and the state health authorities have hindered implementation in the past. Apart from five prisons where condoms were distributed as part of an HIV/AIDS prevention project, by the end of 1997 condom distribution in the state's remaining 37 institutions was undertaken by the guards in a casual manner. "We don't yet have evidence that condoms are being used," says Girao, "or whether they are used more during conjugal visits, between prisoners or are being taken home by the prisoner's family."

A prison programme financed by the World Bank plans to raise awareness among directors of prison systems, provide training for doctors and nurses and prevention workshops for inmates and guards, as well as the production of educational materials such as posters and the distribution of 750,000 condoms. However, the project is limited "because only 15 prisons were interested in proposing a workplan and making available personnel to work in AIDS prevention," says Paulo Junqueira. "We train the professionals and supply the necessary material. But we cannot oblige state governments to demonstrate the political will to change the situation in prisons. As for municipal jails, everything is much more difficult."

Lampadinha and Tereza

There have been a few innovative prison HIV/AIDS prevention programmes. In 1991 the Porto Alegre AIDS Prevention Group (GAPA-Porto Alegre) developed Lampadinha, a 'superhero' prisoner in a comic book who fought against AIDS, as part of a programme of safe sex workshops attended by 3,000 prisoners. The project was less successful outside Porto Alegre, partly because of the use of local slang unfamiliar in the rest of Brazil and partly because of lack of interest by prison governors and a shortage of people to run the project. Although now defunct, Lampadinha served as the seed for *Arpão* (Harpoon), a newspaper written for and by prisoners.

Tereza — prison slang for a rope made of sheets used in escape attempts — is a project created by the Social Health and Orientation Nucleus (NOSS), a Rio de Janeiro-based organisation working with marginalised groups. Between 1991 and 1995 its volunteers reached 6,000 prisoners in 10 institutions with individual counselling, training of prisoners as peer educators, poetry contests, and theatre performances in which the issue of AIDS always featured. NOSS won inmates' confidence. "The fact that the prisoners faithfully attended the workshops, and the relationships we built up with them, suggests that they assimilated the information and adopted safer sex," said Sylvio de Oliveira, former Tereza coordinator. When NOSS workers denounced compulsory testing for HIV and submitted an internal memorandum criticising the prison system, they were expelled from the jails.

Common sense and humanity

It is difficult to come to any conclusion other than that Brazilian prisons are warehouses in which prisoners are treated like animals. The authorities are accomplices in the double punishment to which the prisoners are subjected: the penalty decreed by justice and the penalty imposed by lack of care and the absence of HIV prevention and control. With 60,000 extra places needed, overcrowding is one of the most pressing problems. It could be partly resolved by adopting alternative penalties, such as compensation payments to victims' families, community service and curtailment of civil rights. About 50,000 prisoners could benefit from such measures.

To reduce the spread of HIV, state governments must first admit that sex and drugs are found in prisons. Implementing prevention projects aimed at men who have sex with men, instigating harm-reduction practices, exchanging syringes and distributing condoms is even more necessary. Prevention practices could also be encouraged for conjugal visits. Finally, there should be training of prison personnel and health professionals in prevention and assistance, and prisoners with AIDS should have the same rights to health care as enjoyed by ordinary citizens. It is a question of public health, common sense and humanity.

ACROSS THE BORDER

INTRODUCTION

Since prehistory, war has been waged almost exclusively by men. In recent years women have enrolled in both official armed forces and insurrection movements, but only in a handful of countries have they taken up full combat roles. To all intents and purposes, the military of almost every nation remains a male preserve.

It is therefore not surprising that there is a close overlap between military and masculine values. To be a soldier* is, above all, to be a man — to be strong, brave and aggressive in defence of the community and to accept pain and defeat without complaint. These values continue to be widely promulgated, from Hollywood films such as Rambo *and* Independence Day *to the traditional ceremonies, dances and songs found in almost every popular culture, and the ethos that brings together gangs of young men in large cities across the world.*

A soldier's sexual prowess does not help him fight but is often integral to his self-image. Not only does a man 'prove himself' both on the battlefield and in bed, but the language men use to describe sex is often similar to that of conflict and conquest. Sexual activity increases in war, either on a voluntary basis or in acts of rape. Where armies are undisciplined or encouraged to terrorise, as in the recent conflicts in Bosnia and Rwanda, mass rape may be common. In peacetime the circumstances differ, but soldiers remain keen to have intercourse, and fulfilling that desire places them and their partners at high risk of HIV.

---

* In this chapter, unless otherwise specified, the term 'soldier' refers to any member of the armed forces, including navy and air force personnel, as well as any armed member of an insurrection movement.

Soldiers at risk

Most military personnel are under 35, the most sexually active age group. They leave homes where they interact with both sexes, all ages and a range of values to live only with men who often have limited experience and understanding of the world. Their occupation encourages risk-taking and gives a sense of invulnerability. They either have no regular sexual partners or are separated from them for long periods. Off duty, with money to spend, free from the constraints of their home communities and barracks' discipline, and with inhibitions often loosened by alcohol, they frequently seek sex. They usually do not have to look far: close to camp, in bars, brothels and on the streets, women and sometimes men with financial, emotional and sexual needs of their own are often to be found waiting to meet the soldiers who emerge [1].

Statistics confirm that soldiers are highly sexually active. Studies in the Dutch and US military indicate that 40 to 50 percent of personnel engage in casual sex while on mission. In one survey, 10 percent of this group contracted a sexually transmitted infection (STI) [2]. Data from a number of armies show that soldiers consistently have a higher rate of HIV infection than the general population. Recent surveys have indicated HIV in four percent of recruits from northern Thailand (two percent in the adult population), 22 percent of recruits in the Central African Republic (11 percent in the adult population) and 50 percent of troops in Angola (two percent in the adult population) [3]. Rates are generally highest within navies and armies and lowest in air forces, where the standard of education is higher. The correlation in civilian life between education, age and low HIV prevalence suggests that rates among officers should be lower than amongst their men. This is not always the case, particularly in countries where the status and income associated with being an officer enables them to have intercourse with many women.

A pattern of infection

High rates of HIV among soldiers mirror the prevalence of other STDs, which in peacetime is typically two to five times higher in the military than in the civilian population. (In warfare and times of civil strife, when the attitude 'I might die tomorrow, so I should live today' is common, rates may be 100 times higher than in the general population [4].)

These statistics confirm that even in times of peace, military life heightens the risk that soldiers will contract STDs. When soldiers have a limited choice of sexual partners — because they are far from a city or because the authorities place restrictions on their off-duty life — many men from the same company are likely to have sex with the same women over a period of time; when that company is replaced, the new soldiers have intercourse with those same women. Even if only a small number of soldiers or their partners have a disease at the beginning of this process, frequent sexual activity without a condom will soon cause the disease to spread to others.

The soldiers' next billeting determines who will next contract the disease. As one example, it has been suggested that some personnel in the United Nations peace-keeping force in Cambodia in 1995 contracted a specific sub-type of HIV from the civilian population there [5].

Between men

Although most soldiers contract HIV through sex with women, some will contract the virus through drug injection — almost always before enlisting — or through sex with other men. Little information is available about the extent of sexual activity between soldiers or between soldiers and civilian men. (One of the few studies to research the topic, in Thailand, indicated that 16 percent of recruits had had sex at least once with a man [6].)

While an emotional bond among soldiers as a group is encouraged, sex between men is seen as effeminacy and weakness, and therefore incompatible with military life. With the exception of the armed forces of a few Western countries, soldiers known to have sex with other soldiers or male civilians are almost always punished and usually discharged. Nevertheless, officers in many countries admit off the record that some of their troops have sex with each other or with other men. As discussed in previous chapters, this may be from desire, experimentation or lack of contact with women; it may occasionally be through force. Although those soldiers are at risk of contracting HIV, military policy means that they will almost never receive official advice about how to protect themselves from infection.

In some countries, children, mostly boys, volunteer for or are coerced into fighting forces, particularly insurrection movements. As one commentator points out, even when forced into service children may "see membership of a combative force as the only means of ensuring their survival, as the social fabric of society breaks down and traditional support systems, including their own families, cannot provide for them. Apart from receiving the material means of survival, boy soldiers may meet their need for more intangible forms of nurturing ... through developing a form of father-son relationship with commanding officers" [7]. Relationships with a commanding officer or with older soldiers may become sexual, on either a voluntary or forced basis. In such cases the older man, who may have had considerable sexual experience, is more likely to have HIV or another STD and the younger partner is therefore at high risk of contracting the infection.

Women at risk

In many ways women are more affected by warfare than men. In addition to being the victims of rape and other physical abuse, they constitute more than three in four of the world's refugees [8]. Women also have to cope with the effect of the destruction of family units; they nurse the wounded, care for the orphaned and play a central part in rebuilding shattered communities [9]. At times they are also combatants, with the risk of death and injury that such a role plays. Yet even this is not the full extent of the military impact on women: in both war and peace women, as sexual partners, are directly affected by the actions of soldiers.

Since rates of infection are much higher in the military, those who have sex with soldiers are at greater risk of contracting HIV or other diseases than if their partners were from the general population. Depending on the circumstances, soldiers' sexual partners may or may not be able to protect themselves. Sex workers may demand use of a condom, although a soldier's relative wealth may overcome that demand. Whether during service or after discharge, the wives or long-term partners of soldiers face the same difficulties as other wives in demanding condoms, since many husbands consider it their right to insist on sex without protection.

Soldiers also rape women, children and men [10]. This may be what has been described as 'recreational rape', where individual soldiers decide to have sex irrespective of the wishes of their partner, or systematic mass rape used as an instrument of war. Confirming the existence and extent of mass rape is difficult, particularly since the order is likely to have been verbal and possibly ambiguous, but one study reports systematic rape of women and children by soldiers in over 20 countries across the world in the last 30 years [11].

Whatever the circumstances, victims of rape cannot protect themselves from HIV. Indeed, it has been suggested that the virus itself has been a weapon of war. In 1995 it was reported [12] that women in the Rwandan conflict were deliberately brought to HIV-positive soldiers to be raped. This seems unlikely, since few soldiers would have been aware of their status or announced it to others, but since rates of HIV were very high and rape undoubtedly occurred, it can be assumed that the virus was frequently transmitted through rape at that time.

Military reaction

The institutional implications of high rates of HIV for the military are serious. Loss of members of the ranks to illness and death leads to increased recruitment and training costs for replacements, while loss of officers means the loss of continuity at command level. Lieutenant General D Raghunath (now retired), when director-general of the Indian Armed Forces Medical Services, claimed that prevalence in his country's military was lower than in the general population, yet he commented: "AIDS has made its presence felt in the armed forces.

Combat efficiency will definitely be affected"[13]. Theoreticians suggest that if the situation is serious, there may be a general reduction in preparedness; this may in turn lead to a less stable military.

The armed forces in a number of countries have begun taking steps to reduce the prevalence of HIV. These include the testing of new recruits, which can lead to the exclusion of those discovered to be HIV-positive, and the testing of soldiers in specific circumstances, such as before deployment. Condoms are distributed (by 64 percent of military forces in one survey [14]) and education programmes established. In Zambia, for example, educators include representatives of all ranks, and workshops are aimed at officers, other ranks and soldiers' wives. Other attempts to reduce the spread of HIV include inspecting brothels frequented by the military and demanding regular tests from the women who work there, a strategy which predates AIDS and has included monitoring for gonorrhoea and syphilis. These and other measures, such as prohibiting off-duty soldiers from visiting specific areas or consorting with women who have not been inspected, may reduce the spread of HIV, but some soldiers will still succeed in having intercourse with 'unapproved' partners.

Overall, however, HIV/AIDS prevention programmes in the military are still in the early stages of development, and progress reports have shown little change in the rate at which soldiers contract HIV. Although the armed forces often draw on civilian expertise in devising prevention programmes, the recommendations of civilians are sometimes either poorly understood or ignored. At the Mbarara Military Training Wing in Uganda in January 1997, the names of 114 HIV-positive recruits (11 percent of those tested), including 21 of 27 women recruits, were read out and announced as "medically unfit to join the army" [15]. Greater awareness of the issue both on a national level and through international bodies such as the Civil-Military Alliance to Combat HIV and AIDS may keep such incidents to a minimum in the future. The extent to which insurrection movements also adopt anti-HIV measures is unknown; where there is strict discipline and rape is eschewed as a means of terror, the transmitting of the virus to others may be reasonably contained.

Men at war

Wars vary in their duration, their destructiveness and in the number of civilian casualties they cause. The conflict between Mozambican government troops and the insurrectionist RENAMO movement in the 1980s was characterised by brutality, particularly by the rebels. A third country, Malawi, was drawn in, sending troops into Mozambique to protect its vital railway access to the ocean (the Nacala line).

Hundreds of Malawian troops saw action, with fierce battles at Mtwari, Mamina, Cuamba and other places along the line that they were defending. However, to many young Malawian men the war appeared a heaven-sent opportunity to leave home, earn money and have sex. As such they were typical of inexperienced soldiers across the world who see war as glory and the men who practise war as heroes. In this report Kaulanda Nkosi listens to men and women who shared that first excitement, and looks at the consequences a decade or more later.

MEN, THE MILITARY AND HIV/AIDS IN MALAWI

by Kaulanda Nkosi

Some 40 kilometres west of Lilongwe, the capital of the southern African state of Malawi, Bruno Banda crouches on a tattered mattress in a dark corner of his mother's mud hut. Banda, a 25-year-old soldier, has come home to die. Diagnosed HIV-positive five years ago, he has now developed the symptoms of AIDS: unstoppable diarrhoea, vomiting, general weakness and body pains.

Two weeks ago Rightwell Mwale, another HIV-positive soldier, insisted on being brought back to his home in the next village. But when a visitor asks about him, the villagers do not want to answer. Instead, they exchange furtive glances. From their looks, it is clear that the worst has happened. "He's dead, isn't he?" The villagers nod.

These scenarios are common. In a country now at peace,

the army loses an average of 20 soldiers a month from every rank to AIDS. No one can be certain how they contracted HIV, but the fates of officers and men were sealed as long ago as 1975, when the Portuguese were driven out of their colony Mozambique by guerrillas fighting for their freedom.

A 17-year war

When the Portuguese abandoned the territory, fighting immediately broke out between the rebel movement RENAMO and the new government. For the next 17 years life in Mozambique was disrupted by guerrilla warfare, with RENAMO notorious for attacking villages, destroying infrastructure and terrorising the civilian population.

Malawi, landlocked and dependent on the Mozambican port of Beira for imports and exports, negotiated with the Mozambique government for the construction of a second, shorter railway line to the port of Nacala. The line, completed in 1985, became the target of RENAMO attacks, making it necessary for a joint Malawi-Mozambique military operation for the safe passage of goods, an operation which lasted until 1993. To defend the line, Malawi sent a battalion of 500 soldiers that was replaced every six months.

"Like manna from heaven"

Then, as now, the majority of officers and men recruited by the Malawian army were between 18 and 30 years old, unmarried and therefore with few or no responsibilities. Recruitment was voluntary. Many soldiers were sent to Mozambique immediately after basic training, and most were excited by the thought of going to war. "I had just finished my cadet officer training when I was selected and you can imagine how excited I was," recalls Captain David Majawa. "To me it meant an opportunity to immediately start practising the leadership skills I had learnt." Benson Chikopa was 20 when he was recruited. A primary school drop-out, Chikopa says it was the dream of every Malawian soldier and officer to be posted to Mozambique on military operations. "With such fat allowances [equivalent to US$0.50 a day] we used to enjoy life while there and on our way to and from Mozambique." Chikopa, now 34, has left the army, is HIV-positive and has lost his wife to AIDS.

If the soldiers were happy to see action, so were the women who lived on their transit route. Says Hendrina Naphiri, who runs a small shop at Liwonde, a township on the Nacala line some 70 kilometres from the Mozambique border, "They were quite different from other men. They were not stingy with their money if you had sex with them. If you had a boyfriend among them you were assured of gifts, such as a radio or salt, when they came back from Mozambique. I started the business that I am doing today because of that. It is sad that the operations had to come to an end."

Edith Meleka, a 'freelance' (sex worker), also has fond memories of the soldiers. "They used to make Liwonde lively. They would flood the pubs and beer would flow like manna from heaven." Her cousin, Raphael, comments: "Was there any girl around who did not have a soldier boyfriend? Some of them even had more than one." Apparently resentful, Raphael claims the women became so "stupid" that they even abandoned their local boyfriends on finding a soldier. "There were even cases of married women abandoning their husbands because of soldiers," he recalls.

Asked if she fears that she might have contracted HIV during this time, Edith Meleka replies, "God has given each one of us the day we will die." She admits that several of her friends who befriended soldiers have since died, but she argues that it means nothing more than that their time had come. Fatima Mbewe from Ntaja, another township on the

Nacala line, points out that most women who had sexual relationships with the soldiers had seen no threat. "There was no AIDS at that time," Mbewe says. In fact, the first case in Malawi was diagnosed the year the Nacala operation started, but it was several years before the authorities openly acknowledged that the disease posed a problem.

Effromina, Maria Zinya and Gloria

Twenty years ago Cuamba was a small, sleepy town on the Mozambique side of the Nacala line. Today it is a hive of activity which owes much of its growth to the arrival of Mozambican and Malawian soldiers who came to defend the line in 1987. According to local shop owner Festino Mawayi, most of the shops, bars and resthouses were built at that time. "Resthouses became one of the most lucrative businesses. They were ideal for a soldier who wanted 'a quick one' with a woman and dash back to the camp before his bosses discovered he was absent. In such a situation," Mawayi adds with a chuckle, "you can charge anything." Maria Maluwa remembers living in a house in the regional capital of Nampula where she and other sex workers frequently entertained Malawian soldiers. "Each time they arrived in the city they used to come to our place and we would eat with them. We really used to enjoy ourselves," she recalls nostalgically.

A Malawian captain recalls how exciting it was to make return trips to Mozambique, because it gave soldiers the opportunity of meeting up with women they had got to know previously. "The names of women who were popular at this time were Effromina, Maria Zinya and Gloria. It was the dream of every Malawian soldier to sleep with these women. They were said to be very sweet in bed." The attitude of many men towards Mozambique and its women can be summed up in a song that many of the men sang:

I will not go to Mozambique
I fear the waters will sweep me away
Your buttocks, your breasts have captured my imagination
No, I will not go to Mozambique

Antonio Fernandez, a senior officer in the Mozambican army who enlisted in 1988, contends that no threat of disciplinary action can stop soldiers from sneaking out of camp to meet their girlfriends. "It is true that during the war soldiers had less freedom to walk around than they have today, but on the few occasions they were allowed or sneaked out they could have contracted HIV." At the time, Fernandez points out, few people had heard of AIDS and those who had heard about it "felt AIDS was for homosexuals in America and Ugandans in Africa. Of course, we were to learn that it was in Malawi."

Joe Nasala, who has since left the army and is now HIV-positive, has no regrets. "Everybody had girlfriends there. We all went out to drink and have a good time." On average, he claims, most Malawian soldiers had sex with 10 or more different women a month. Married, with two children, Nasala regularly sent some money to his wife, but spent most of it on beer and women. "You see, soldiers like to conquer. The more women you take to bed the more you feel like a real man. We never thought about AIDS. Our only fear as we drank and had sex was a sudden attack from RENAMO rebels."

Soldiers in the Mozambican army were less fortunate than their allies. "Those people [Malawians] had money and they could drink and buy all the women around," Mawayi says. "Our soldiers couldn't compete with them." Graciano Mende, an ex-combatant with the Mozambican armed forces, echoes his comments. "They used to have more money than us. They were paid regularly, while our pay was erratic. And because of this they were popular with our women."

Fear and violence

Mozambican women may have welcomed the Malawian army, but they often had cause to fear their own compatriots. Acts of terror by RENAMO were common, carried out to undermine confidence in the Mozambique government, punish its supporters, plunder for food and pressgang able-bodied young men into their forces. The army was less brutal because it wanted to restore the population's confidence in the government, although it sometimes terrorised villages suspected of collaborating with the insurrectionists. In comparison, the Malawian soldiers were more disciplined. "Morale was high among our soldiers because they had everything they could dream about," says one Malawian officer. "We made sure we put their welfare first so they had no reason to terrorise the civilian population."

Gosta Almanda is one of the few Mozambicans who fought on both sides in the war. After serving FRELIMO for several years, he, his wife and three-year-old son were abducted by RENAMO and compelled to fight. Now demobilised, he has a permanent limp from a bullet wound in the thigh.

Almanda explains that it was not wise for soldiers in either army to overindulge sexually, for fear that the women would betray them to the enemy. "You see, in this war it was not easy to tell who was on your side. Besides, suppose you are sitting drinking in a bar and having fun when the enemy surrounds you. What happens? You all perish."

Yet there were times when the soldiers had as much sex as they wanted, irrespective of the women's wishes. Almanda relates a typical experience as a RENAMO soldier: "One day we entered a village and axed to death all the old people and invalids, took away the girls and boys and raped women in front of their own husbands and parents-in-law." (Married couples often share a home with the husband's parents.)

Almanda's claims that such incidents were commonplace

are supported by others. There are stories of women fetching water and firewood who were raped by rampaging soldiers. Some of these women disappeared without trace, while most of those who survived are too shocked and ashamed to talk about their experiences.

Ellena Amisi counts herself lucky because though some of her friends were brutally assaulted, she was never a victim. "My friend Josephina was raped by 12 RENAMO soldiers who abducted her, but she managed to escape. It was a terrible time for us women," she recalls with a shudder and asks, "Can we talk about something else now?" Josephina herself has since disappeared and neither her friends nor family know where she is.

The aftermath

Most Malawian officers who led troops in Mozambique do not want to be reminded of their exploits while they were there. "My friend, let's not talk about the sexual behaviour of soldiers while on service in Mozambique. What would you have done if you had been there?" one officer asks. When pressed, however, he admits that most of his contemporaries have either died from AIDS-related diseases or are terminally ill. Exact statistics are not available. More than half the officers and men interviewed for this article said that living with HIV/AIDS was worse than being at war, especially because they did not know if their girlfriends had contracted the disease.

It is difficult to tell how many soldiers contracted or passed on HIV during the Mozambique campaign and how many became HIV-positive later, but the army today is badly affected. One unpublished study shows that the military and police have the highest rate of infection in the country. Army medical staff say their offices are inundated with requests for recommendation for early retirement from soldiers with HIV/AIDS. "Most of such requests come from the terminally ill," says one senior clinical officer, although on occasion "we also receive requests from soldiers who have just been told they have the virus."

Although it is not easy to determine the extent to which AIDS has affected the military in Mozambique, soldiers there are dying of HIV-related diseases. "I know some of my own colleagues have apparently died of AIDS," says Captain Fernandez. "Since they say that HIV takes about 10 years to develop into AIDS, we can assume, with some degree of exactitude, that these people were infected during the war."

First steps

Despite the severity of the AIDS epidemic that is now officially recognised in Malawi (in some cities one adult in three is HIV-positive), the army seems reluctant to address the problem within its own ranks. The issue was first discussed in January 1996, when a workshop for senior army officers concluded that some military regulations, such as the ban on officers and men marrying in the first nine months after their basic training, did not promote good health. (Only unmarried men can join the army.) Three months later a workshop bringing together civilians and the military led to a number of policy recommendations intended to reduce the risk of soldiers contracting HIV. Suggestions included lifting the ban on marriage after training and allowing spouses to accompany soldiers and officers on long tours of duty.

It is clear that further steps are needed. In 1997 an army officer responsible for developing AIDS prevention policy claimed that many senior officers knew or suspected they had contracted HIV themselves but were afraid of drawing attention to the issue. The officer pointed out that there had been strong criticism of senior staff by junior officers, who felt that neglect of the issue was putting their own lives at risk. Lack of action by the army leadership has led to uncertainty in the ranks. Soldiers recently vandalised the offices of the *Daily Times* newspaper, after it quoted a statement in a report by a World Bank assessment team about the high incidence of HIV in the Malawian military.

In Mozambique, where UNAIDS estimates that 14 percent of adults have contracted HIV, the attitude of many people to the AIDS epidemic is even less open. In Maputo, the capital, a senior army officer threatened me with arrest if I continued researching the topic, though other contacts were more helpful.

Even today many Mozambicans are reluctant to face the reality of AIDS. The barman in the Kusuuando Hotel in Tete, 800 kilometres north-west of Beira, says locals rarely ask for Jeito condoms. "If you see someone asking for a condom, you know they are a foreigner," he says. "Very often a week will pass without a single packet of Jeito being sold."

A New Lease on Life

INTRODUCTION

In 1998 it was estimated that more than 30 million people around the world were living with HIV, 17 million of whom were men. Most are unaware of their infection. Some who are aware remain symptom-free for years, their way of life continuing almost unchanged. Others learn of their status only when they fall ill with an opportunistic infection. They may recover or they may find that this is the first stage in a gradual and relentless deterioration in their health.

Two types of treatment are available: drugs that attack opportunistic infections, such as tuberculosis, irrespective of whether the individual has HIV; and antivirals, such as protease inhibitors, which prevent HIV from reproducing. Antivirals have offered a new lease of life to many in the West who expected early death, although some find their bodies are unable to tolerate the severe side-effects. In the developing world increasing numbers of people have access to a range of antivirals, but the cost is far beyond the means of most individuals and health services. This means that for most men and women in the foreseeable future, HIV will lead to premature death.

Yet because it may not lead to AIDS for many years, in the short term the physical impact of HIV is less important than the knowledge of having contracted the virus. Some react with despair, others with apparent indifference, yet none can ignore the fact that their life has changed radically. How men and women respond to this shift depends on a number of factors, but critical is the support that they receive from family, friends and –

increasingly — organisations dedicated to helping those with HIV.

In countries, particularly in the West, where most of those who have contracted HIV are men who have sex with men, the strongest support groups appear to be for men. In countries where both men and women are affected, particularly in sub-Saharan Africa, it seems that women have the strongest networks, both before and after diagnosis. Although little research has been undertaken in this area, it appears that this situation leads to men in the North, but women in the South, surviving longer with AIDS.

As Satya Sivaraman reports, this analysis is reflected — at least in part — in Thailand, where one in every 50 adults has HIV. Strong government efforts to reduce the spread of the virus, coupled with the work of non-governmental organisations (NGOs) in both prevention and care, have reduced the stigma and increased awareness of the disease throughout the country. Nevertheless, stigmatisation still occurs, and for that and other reasons it remains difficult for many men to accept the fact that they are HIV-positive.

LIVING WITH HIV/AIDS IN THAILAND
by Satya Sivaraman

When doctors at a Bangkok hospital informed Samran, a young interior designer who had just turned 30, that his tuberculosis was a symptom of AIDS, he was shattered. Convinced that death was just days or weeks away, he quit his job, packed his bags and went off to spend his last days in a Buddhist monastery in Lopburi, 150 kilometres from Bangkok.

"I thought I was the first man in Thailand to have AIDS," he recalls. The first cases of the disease had been detected only five years earlier, in 1984, and Samran had heard of very few people who were even HIV-positive. He had, however, seen enough government information posters of people with advanced AIDS to convince him that he neither wanted nor would be able to continue living.

To his surprise, he discovered over 200 other people with HIV living in the monastery, all with the same intention: to die. The pointlessness of so many people waiting for death sparked Samran's desire to fight back, however painful living might prove to be. Nine years later he is healthy and robust, with no traces of tuberculosis or any other opportunistic disease. He is also extremely busy, working for the New Life Friends Association, an organisation he and others with the virus set up in 1995 in the northern city of Chiang Mai.

Samran is well known and is often referred to by local health activists as the "superstar" of people with HIV. He is, however, not unique. Thanks to his example and the work of organisations such as New Life, thousands of Thai men and women are learning to cope with their HIV status, fight discrimination and lead normal, dignified lives. Their attitude can be summed up in Samran's words: "Nobody lives for ever, so why all this fuss about people who are HIV-positive or have AIDS dying?"

Testing positive

The way in which men and women learn they have HIV and respond to the diagnosis reflects the culture in which they live. Despite frequenting sex workers, most Thai men do not have regular check-ups for sexually transmitted diseases. They discover they have the virus only after they fall sick and are treated for symptoms of AIDS or unrelated ailments. This behaviour, says Natee Teerarojanapongs, one of the country's best known AIDS activists, stems from the common belief that as long as 'luck' is on a man's side, nothing bad can happen to him.

Piyaporn, 26, a native of Mae Rim, who used to work as a bartender at a five-star hotel in the island resort of Koh

Samui, discovered he was HIV-positive during hospital treatment for injuries sustained in a motorcycle accident. His wife, whom he had married a month before the accident, also tested positive. Sak, 33, a native of Chiang Rai in the north of country, "had a check-up in February 1995 after developing symptoms of fever and tuberculosis, and tested positive." Married in 1990, with a daughter, Sak was lucky to find support and understanding from his wife, who does not have HIV; he believes that he contracted the virus from sex workers prior to his marriage.

Secrecy

Most HIV-positive men in Thailand try to hide their status from both family and friends. According to HIV/AIDS activists, educated urban men are often secretive as they are afraid of discrimination and of 'losing face' and status if they admit they have the virus. Rural men appear relatively more open about the problem.

"I didn't tell anyone about testing HIV-positive for more than a year, until I fell sick repeatedly and had to inform my friends. My parents learnt about my condition through other sources and were very sad," recalls Pong, 25, a video cameraman in Chiang Mai. He discovered his status when he was about to get married; having read government posters urging men to visit the doctor before marriage, he asked for an HIV test. Pong, who believes that he contracted the virus from a nightclub waitress, says that he did not immediately tell anyone because he was afraid of losing his job and was worried about the impact of the news on his parents.

When they do decide to confide, Thai men usually inform close family members, such as their parents, wife or siblings. Depending on the reaction, they then tend to tell their close friends and try to win acceptance from them. "The first person I informed about testing HIV-positive was my brother, and then I told my parents. My father was very upset but he and the rest of the family have now accepted me. Now even my friends in the village accept me and often invite me home and ask me to their parties," says Anan, a 32-year-old construction worker in Baan Huarin village, 35 kilometres from Chiang Mai. Pichet Saikhamya, another construction worker, says he started talking about his condition with other HIV-positive people in his village two years ago: "Most of my neighbours and friends initially did not accept me, but with the passage of time they have begun to do so."

Fear of abandonment

Many Thai women complain that men of every social class refuse to tell their spouses about their HIV status because of their big egos and fear of humiliation, says Phimjai Inthamun, coordinator of the Community Health Centre at Mae Rim. This silence is the primary cause of the rapid spread of HIV among housewives in Thailand.

"Some men are known to have deliberately passed on the HIV virus to their wives because they are afraid of being left alone. Fear of being abandoned by their family also plays a big role in men not revealing their status," says Dr Usa Duongsa of AIDSNET, a Chiang Mai-based NGO. However, Duongsa qualifies this comment by noting that far more men abandon HIV-positive wives than women abandon HIV-positive husbands. Tradition, she points out, encourages women to stay and look after their sick husbands. Women whose husbands leave them tend to return to their parents or scrape a living to look after their children.

Duongsa believes that more and more women are mustering the courage to question the behaviour of their husbands and insist on the use of condoms during marital sex, but the majority still quietly accept whatever happens as bad luck, in line with the Buddhist notion of *karma* (destiny).

"Men lose heart easily"

"I was so shocked that I thought everything was finished. I really felt very sorry," says Sak, quoted earlier. Ironically, the 'superior' status of men in Thai society is not always reflected in an ability to cope with HIV. While bravado frequently characterises their behaviour in everyday life, many men who test positive for the virus appear to lose the will to live. No figures are available, but AIDS workers and media reports indicate that a significant number of men with HIV commit suicide or let their health deteriorate. Activists such as Phimjai Inthamun suggest that suicides among HIV-positive men could be 10 times higher than amongst women in a similar condition.

"In the context of the ordinary Thai household, men usually get infected much earlier than women," Phimjai points out, "but we notice that, on average, men with HIV also tend to die faster than women because they lose heart easily. Women live on because they are often motivated by the desire to look after their children and other members of the family, whereas men think only of themselves." Phimjai, who tested positive in 1993 after her husband fell ill with AIDS, runs a counselling and hospice service for 400 people with HIV in over 80 villages in the Mae Rim area. She claims that men with the virus tend to neglect themselves more than do women; they lack discipline and continue to drink, smoke and indulge in sexual activities, all of which may hasten their death.

Ree, 32, a shopworker in Chiang Mai, tested positive in February 1993, when her husband fell sick and the couple had blood tests at a local hospital. Ree is sure that her husband, an engineer who died in 1995, contracted HIV from sex workers while travelling around the country for his work. "I felt very sad and upset and at first wanted to kill myself because I thought even my son, who was just two years old at that time, would be HIV-positive. But when a check-up revealed that he was not affected, I changed my mind and mustered the will to live and bring up the child." Now Ree works as a volunteer for the New Life Friends Association. She admits to being angry with her husband for giving her HIV, but feels that widespread patronage of sex workers cannot be blamed on men alone.

"Most people with HIV who die quickly do so because of negative thinking. Cancer caused by smoking or other reasons is more dangerous than AIDS. What we require is positive thinking," says Somboon Suprasert, a trained public health specialist and prominent businesswoman. Somboon is a major fund raiser for HIV/AIDS groups in Chiang Mai and director of a centre for people with HIV that teaches 'life skills', using a holistic approach to tackle their problems. Not all men agree that their reactions to HIV are more negative than women's. Pichet, mentioned earlier, claims that, "I could accept my fate more quickly than [my wife] because I thought that I was the person to blame for contracting HIV in the first place."

Sex and manhood

Diagnosis of HIV may have a strong impact on a man's sense of masculinity. Pichet says that, "When I first learned about my HIV status, my wife and I stopped having sex. I was so sad that I couldn't think of having sex. But after five or six months I began again. We always use condoms." Prathuan had a similar experience: "When I learned about my HIV status, I was still single and believed I had lost my masculinity. After a year, I became stronger in my mind. Meditation at the temple also helped me recover my morale."

Pornchai says, "At first when I learned about my HIV status I stopped sleeping with my wife. I tried to control my mind a lot but I realised that I still needed sex. All the time I blamed myself. At that time I felt that I had lost my masculinity because I could not satisfy my wife. Later, when my wife also discovered she was HIV-positive, we resumed our sex life, though with a lot of precautions. Now we have a normal sex life."

But Sonchai's wife is HIV-negative and he has a different response. "Since I learnt that I am HIV-positive, I have not had sex, even with my wife. I'm not afraid of having sex, but I don't want anybody to get HIV from me. I don't think I have lost face or lost my masculinity. My wife accepts and understands me and has never put me in a situation where I would lose face."

"Employers turn us away"

Men may also face loss of income. Pichet started working in his family's shop when his health stopped him doing heavy labour. "My income decreased by 30 percent after I left my job. My wife was employed in a computer shop and she continued working for three years without telling her employers. She resigned after some symptoms of AIDS started appearing and one of her colleagues found out. We managed to save about 100,000 baht (US$2,600) before giving up our jobs, but we spent all the money looking after our health, especially on buying medicines."

Prathuan also left his job as a construction worker and now works for his parents on their land. His wife, who is also HIV-positive, works with them and they have been able to save some money for their son. Sonchai stopped working as a barber soon after learning he had HIV. "Many customers were afraid of coming to me for fear of contracting HIV from my equipment." He, too, now works with his parents, although his wife still earns money as a tailor.

Both Adul and his wife have been forced to give up work. They live off relatives, who supply them with food. Pornchai, another construction worker, has temporarily stopped work. "My wife's health has deteriorated very quickly and she has had to go into hospital. I'll go back to work again soon. The money we get every month is very little, so we are trying to economise. If we do not get any financial support from [New Life or a similar organisation] I will work as a labourer until my symptoms appear again. It's very difficult to find a job these days because many employers turn us away when they know we are HIV-positive."

A new lease on life

Despite all the economic, social and personal problems of people with HIV, a growing number believe that the best form of defence is to go on the offensive. "People who are HIV-positive are normal people and I want them to be convinced of that," says Samran, whose New Life Friends Association now has nearly 6,000 members in six northern provinces. The organisation acts as a magnet for people with HIV in other parts of the country who come to it for advice, moral support and expertise on tackling their medical and social problems. The presence of New Life and other organisations has provided a major morale boost to people with HIV, who say that discussing common problems with others with the virus gives them a sense of belonging and revives their desire to lead normal lives.

Apart from its morale-raising role, New Life teaches personal and medical care and advises on the use of Western and indigenous herbal medicines. This counselling work is done at the New Life offices in several towns, as well as by volunteers visiting people at home. At times the organisation also musters financial support from various sources to help those with HIV in dire need of money and material help. Many of those who first come to New Life for help on learning they are HIV-positive become volunteers for the organisation.

"To know that one is not alone and also to be able to help other people in trouble has a very calming effect on my mind, and Samran's group has given me both," says Pong, who came to New Life after hearing about it at a government-run clinic. There is similar praise for other organisations working on HIV/AIDS in northern Thailand. "Thanks to the volunteers at the Mae Rim Community Health Centre, I got the courage to live on. I want to survive and not worry too much about the future and also be of help to other HIV-positive people," says Piyaporn. Since quitting his job as a bartender in Koh Samui and returning home, Piyaporn has been learning painting, sculpture and silk-screen printing at a government-run institute in Chiang Mai, which he says he enjoys a great deal.

"I would like to get back to my export business, work very hard and provide for my daughter's future," says Sak, whose wife and three-year-old daughter often travel to visit him in Chiang Mai from their village near Chiang Rai. Though he wants to live alone away from his family for fear that people may discriminate against his daughter, Sak says he feels like a perfectly normal person, except that sometimes his health does not permit him to work as much as he wants.

Pichet and his wife, who spent all their savings on their health, have got together with other HIV-positive people in their village to work on a range of income-generating projects. He points out that some of them get 500 baht (US$38) a month from the government and 'seed money' from the Red Cross with which to start their own businesses.

Children

Children, or lack of them, figure prominently in the lives of many men with HIV. Pichet says that he and his wife learned that they had the virus when they decided to take the test before having a child. "But after learning of our HIV status, we had to give up our plans. We were very sad. It took me a year to get over not being able to have a child. The doctor advised us to adopt a child, but I don't want to do that." Adul Boonmasom says that "the only child we had was born in poor health and died at the age of 11 months. Since both [my wife and I] are HIV-positive, we have no plans for more children."

Other men are luckier. Prathuan Deja and his wife are both HIV-positive; she already had a son, who is HIV-negative, when they married. "My wife and I worry a lot about the future of our son. We have asked my parents to adopt him as their own child and bring him up in future, if necessary. I have made a will leaving him all my property." Sonchai Saitha, the barber, has a three-year-old son who is also HIV-negative. "He is too young to know [that Sonchai has HIV]. One problem we have is that other children of his age have been told by their parents that they might get HIV from me and my child, so he doesn't have many friends to play with in the neighbourhood or at the nursery school. I want him to study as much as possible and get a good job, but I haven't been able to prepare anything for his education because I have no money and no support from anywhere."

Combating discrimination

Though in the initial years of the epidemic people affected by HIV were discriminated against by neighbours, friends and sometimes even family members, over the years attitudes have changed. "Some of my close friends stopped eating or even drinking water at my house and were very reluctant to invite me home after learning that I was HIV-positive," recalls Ree. But since her family accepted her and came out into the open about her condition, discrimination has diminished.

It is to help prevent such incidents that people with HIV have set up so many groups. Experts say that Thailand could become a model for developing countries in terms of generating action from within local communities and by those directly affected by the pandemic.

The fight against discrimination is helped by the increasing number of people who refuse to hide behind their HIV status but treat it like any other disease. Such self-confidence plays a key role in helping people without the virus understand that there is nothing mysterious and shameful about it. Organisations such as New Life also play an important role in educating the public about the medical facts, through campaigns in schools, universities and village community centres.

Many men with HIV say that discrimination is not too severe, and is usually based on misplaced fears of contracting HIV through casual contact. "My friends know now that they are not going to become HIV-positive by shaking hands or sharing food and water with me," says Pong. Instances of villagers ostracising or behaving violently towards people with HIV are rare. "So many families have been affected by HIV that it is becoming impossible to discriminate. The government has changed its earlier strategy of propagating ugly pictures of people in advanced stages of AIDS, which were meant to frighten people into changing their sexual behaviour. It is now taking a more positive approach," says Dr Chavalit Natpratan of the Ministry of Health.

Nevertheless, some hostility persists. One highly publicised violent incident occurred in 1996, when residents of a locality in Bangkok were suspected of organising a grenade attack on an HIV/AIDS counselling centre, which they were afraid would attract patients to their area.

In the workplace

Although Thailand has no special law to protect employees with HIV, their rights are usually protected by labour laws framed before the advent of AIDS which prohibit blood tests of prospective employees and ban arbitrary dismissal on grounds of poor health. HIV/AIDS workers say that although most employers in Thailand are accommodating, some reject candidates with the virus or even dismiss existing employees, using poor performance or lack of qualifications as an excuse.

"Companies which discriminate against people with HIV do so out of ignorance, but the number of cases of discrimination has come down drastically since the early days of the epidemic," says Amphai Sheehan, managing director of the Amphai Institute of Hair Design in Chiang Mai, which runs beauty parlours, a fitness centre and a cosmetics plant. Some of the Institute's nearly 100 employees are HIV-positive; there is no discrimination and they are given special medical allowances to help pay for their treatment. "We should approach the problems as if everybody is HIV-positive instead of treating affected people as being isolated cases," Amphai says.

Though few employers have as positive an attitude as Amphai, the general level of awareness about the pandemic among companies has increased considerably in recent years, thanks to the work of HIV/AIDS education groups. Indeed, many business organisations such as Thai Farmers Bank and the Siam Cement conglomerate contribute financially to groups working with people with HIV.

The centre of the community

Buddhism is the national religion and a major effort to help people with HIV aims to get the country's many Buddhist monks involved in the task. Begun in 1997 with funds from the UN Children's Fund (UNICEF), the project is reaching out to monasteries throughout northern Thailand.

"The temple is the centre of the community so monks have a powerful role to play," says Lawrence Maund, a Buddhism scholar who is coordinator of the project. Millions of boys and girls study in monasteries and receive moral instruction as part of the daily curriculum. Many of the boys later become monks themselves, either on a temporary basis or for the rest of their lives. Maund points out that

HIV/AIDS educators have spent little or no time working with monasteries, and their involvement could unleash tremendous social forces.

Though some senior clergy have traditionally frowned on discussion of HIV/AIDS issues by monks, the project has drawn enthusiastic response from younger monks, many of whom have seen family members and friends die of AIDS. Several monasteries in northern Thailand now run meditation centres, counselling services and income-generating activities for people affected by HIV.

A number of monasteries, such as Wat Mai Huay Sai-Suthep in Chiang Mai, provide care for people with HIV who have no homes or who are dying. "We do not have enough funds or expertise to provide advanced medical treatment to patients, but they find a peaceful place to spend their last days," says Phra Phonthep Dhammagaruko, director of the Friends For Life Centre at the monastery.

Maintaining morale

A severe downturn in the Thai economy began in 1997, a recession that at the time of writing sees no sign of ending. Many HIV/AIDS organisations are concerned that this will lead to a cut in government spending on medical care for affected people, as well as reduced funding for NGOs. The prospect of large-scale unemployment could also deprive people with HIV of their regular incomes.

"More than medical care, what people with HIV need most is high morale, and it will be a tough task for us to try and help them maintain that in the current economic situation," says an activist with the New Life Friends Association. Yet given the determination that many of these groups have shown, even this task may not be beyond them.

"The HIV epidemic, more than any other recent phenomenon, has made us aware of the need to concentrate on quality of life and not on mere prolongation of life. Peace of mind takes priority over everything else and once that is achieved, magically other problems like health and even economic well-being are taken care of by themselves," says Phra Greg Dassana, a Canadian Buddhist monk working on meditation techniques for treating HIV patients. For men living with HIV, the message is also to learn from their female counterparts who, by managing their stress better and struggling on for the sake of their children and other family members, are showing that having the infection does not mean either instant death or a painful existence.

TO MARK MY TIME ON EARTH

INTRODUCTION

Most men either are or wish to become fathers, for reasons which are not always consciously understood or expressed. Depending on the culture and circumstances of the family in which they grow up, children perpetuate the family name; they provide additional labour to work on the family's land or supplement its income in other ways; in later life they are responsible for looking after aged parents. They provide proof of a man's virility and a legacy to the world after his death. Last but not least, they are a source of pleasure and pride.

The importance of fathers

If men need children, children need fathers. Apart from matrilineal societies, where the maternal uncle takes the role, the father is usually the most influential adult male in a child's life. However, while mothers are almost always present for their children, taking care of their physical, financial and emotional needs, fathers' involvement in their children's upbringing varies. Many men are absent for long periods, some are abusive and others are unaware that they are fathers, having conceived with women whom they never meet again.

Responsibility for the lack of parenting skills lies with society as much as with individual men; one review of 186 cultures reports that in only two percent do fathers have "regular close relationships" with their children during infancy, and only five percent do so when their children are in early childhood [1]. As Patricia Burke of the

Jamaican National AIDS Committee points out, boys "are not taught to be fathers" [2]. In recent years, while some men have become more involved with the raising of their children, many others have been distanced from their offspring by such factors as divorce, economic migration, imprisonment and the decision of some women to become single mothers. These factors, plus the death of men through accident, war and civil strife, have led to a worldwide increase in the percentage of households headed by women.

Men have greater earning power but contribute less of their income to their children's well-being than do women [3]. For a child, however, a father's positive emotional involvement may be even more important than his financial support. Studies show that infants initially prefer their mothers, but they become attached to their fathers by the end of the first year of life, even if the fathers spend relatively little time with them, and a father's involvement contributes greatly to a child's intellectual, social and emotional development. This is not a one-way process: men who take responsibility for their children's welfare frequently express the importance of their attachment [4].

By default or design

Men become fathers in different circumstances, with poorer, less educated men tending both to begin their sexual lives earlier and not to use family planning techniques. In Latin America many young, unmarried men become fathers by default. Some deny paternity or otherwise refuse to take responsibility for the well-being of the child and its mother. Where the father-to-be is willing to share responsibility for the pregnancy, crucial decisions are often left to the mother, such as whether to insist on marriage, to bring up the child without the father's involvement, to offer the child for adoption or to abort, depending on the options available in her culture. Some young men who recognise paternity find it difficult to adjust to a status for which they are not prepared: "The only thing I said was, 'Well, I'll get married,' but I didn't know what I was saying, 'I'm going to be a father,' but I didn't know what that meant either.'" Others react positively: "The fact of being a father ... is something beautiful. My son has filled my life in many ways, has given me the strength to keep working and studying. I want to give him everything in the future" [5].

It is when men reach their mid-twenties that they begin to want to plan parenthood. In theory the decision as to whether to attempt to conceive a child depends on the agreement of both partners; in practice this is much more common among the middle class than when both partners are poor and have little or no education. In such a situation there is often no discussion and no contraception is used or, occasionally, men take the decision to limit the family size. In some countries, however, where there is widespread access to contraceptives, husbands may agree to their use or wives may take them without their partner's knowledge.

After fatherhood

The long incubation period during which HIV presents no symptoms means that many men learn they have the virus only when their youngest child is diagnosed with AIDS. In a very few cases, the child will have contracted HIV from an infected blood transfusion or a non-sterile needle. Almost always, diagnosis in the child means that the mother is HIV-positive too. Often she will have contracted the virus from the father.

Some men initially deny that they were the first to contract HIV, placing severe strain on relations between the parents and older children who may be affected by their disagreements. "Men often feel guilty about the situation but cannot express it," says Helen Cormann, who has worked with AIDS-affected low-income families in Guatemala. "They can't tell their wives and children they had sex outside the marriage, although the women almost always knew." Zimbabwean commentator Marvellous Mhloyi points out that this situation can affect the whole family: "Conflict heightens between the spouses and children notice the deterioration of their parents' relationship as their sick sibling moves closer to death" [6]. When they eventually accept the news, fathers must then face the possibility that their own illness and death may prevent them from supporting their remaining offspring throughout childhood.

Before fatherhood

As more young men become tested before they start a family, those who learn they are HIV-positive are faced with the possibility of transmitting the virus to their female partner, if she is still HIV-negative, and to a future child. As discussed below, men can become fathers without transmitting the virus to their partner, although this is difficult to achieve and is not guaranteed.

Irrespective of the father's serostatus (whether or not he has the virus), if the mother is HIV-negative, the child will also be HIV-negative. If she is HIV-positive, the child has a 25 to 40 percent chance of also contracting the virus, a rate which falls to about 10 percent if the mother takes zidovudine (AZT) [7]. This means that most children born to seropositive mothers do not contract HIV. However, the prognosis for those who do contract the virus is not good. Of new-borns with HIV, 80 percent develop symptoms of AIDS before they are four. Nonetheless, to many potential parents the risk of a child contracting HIV may be of little importance if they live in a community with a high incidence of malnutrition and other childhood diseases. As discussed below, it is often of much greater importance to both mother and father to leave a child to posterity.

Avoiding risk, achieving conception

Whether or not HIV-positive men discuss the question of fatherhood depends on a range of factors, including education and ease in discussing the issue. Most men and women with the virus are unaware of the fact or convince themselves they are HIV-negative. Where both partners know they have HIV, condoms may not be necessary to prevent transmission of the virus if the wife received the infection from her husband. If both have been faithful there is no risk of introducing a second strain of HIV which would exacerbate the pressure on her immune system. If she contracted the virus from another person, however, condoms should be used when pregnancy is not the goal of intercourse, to prevent 'reinfection'.

Men who know they have HIV while their wives are HIV-

negative are faced with the dilemma that condoms reduce the risk of transmitting the infection to their wives but prevent the pregnancy which both partners may desire. In fact, using condoms at all times except when the woman is at her most fertile period allows the possibility of conception while reducing the risk of the mother and future child contracting the disease. (Men who are HIV-negative but whose wives have HIV can minimise the risk of contracting the virus in the same manner.) For most couples, however, poverty, lack of access to information and the circumstances in which sex takes place means that this combined method may not be available.

Children affected

"Women with HIV are concerned for the future of their children from the start," says Helen Cormann of her experience in Guatemala. "Men with HIV are more concerned with themselves, until they fall ill. Then they want to leave something behind for their children."

Children whose parents are HIV-positive but who themselves do not have the virus can be affected by the disease in many ways. They are more likely to be directly affected by the illness and death of their mother, for usually she is the one who ensures that they are fed, clothed, sheltered and educated to the best of the family's ability. If she is incapacitated, their nutrition is likely to suffer, they are less likely to go to school and they lose the emotional stability essential to a good childhood.

If he lives with the family, a father's illness and death can also be traumatic. His income may be necessary for the family's well-being and his illness will divert the mother's attention and perhaps take time away from income-generating activities. If both are ill, children may be forced to care for their parents at an age when they are still emotionally vulnerable and expect to be cared for themselves. If orphaned, children may find themselves cared for by elderly or distant relatives who are unable or uninterested in properly assuming the task; some children end up living on the streets, the source of many dangers not found in the parental home.

Looking forward

While there have been many studies of the impact of HIV on families [8], few have looked at the topic of men, fatherhood and HIV. This paper was commissioned by Panos to encourage research into this particular area; many moral, economic, medical and other questions have been omitted or only touched on here.

Nevertheless, as it is only in recent years that reproductive health organisations have made greater efforts to involve men in planning their families, it is time for organisations working in AIDS to look at the relationship between men, HIV and fatherhood. This may not only lead more men to protect themselves and their partners from the virus, but may result in more men taking greater responsibility for the children they help to conceive. Different language may also help. As one family planning expert points out, "What is phrased as a responsibility or duty can in many cases also be proposed as a right. Stating that men have a right to care for their children, for example, offers an entirely different approach to the male target audience" [9].

Ivory Coast

Nowhere has the impact of HIV on families been as deeply felt as in sub-Saharan Africa. There, UNAIDS reports, 20 million adults and one million children have contracted the virus and a further eight million children have lost one or both parents to AIDS. The Ivory Coast (also known by its French name of Côte d'Ivoire) is particularly badly affected, with one in 10 adults HIV-positive. While the question of mother-child transmission has been widely discussed, and zidovudine for pregnant mothers is beginning to become available, the question of fatherhood and HIV has been confined to groups of men and women living with the virus. That situation may be about to change, as Hubert N'Goran Kouadio – himself a father with HIV – reports.

HIV/AIDS AND FATHERHOOD IN THE IVORY COAST

by Hubert N'Goran Kouadio

"I tested positive five years ago. I have a partner who tested negative. Since then our preoccupation has been whether to have a child or not," says Ettienne Tape Bi, a founding member of Lumière Action (Action Light), a non-governmental organisation (NGO) formed to promote the interests of people living with HIV. "Our concern is the future of our child after I am dead. If I am working I could take the gamble, but I have been unemployed since I tested positive, because no company wants to employ me."

Tape Bi's situation is not unique. According to Ivory Coast estimates, about 800,000 people in a population of 14 million are believed to be living with HIV, with both sexes equally affected. Some 400,000 children have lost one or both parents to AIDS, while at least 15,000 children a year are born with the disease [10].

For the first few years after the epidemic's appearance in the country, the general reaction was of fear and denial. With little or no information and little help from NGOs, people with AIDS hid themselves at home or returned to their village to die. Only since the early 1990s, when more NGOs became active and people with HIV began appearing on television and other media, has Ivorian society begun to accept that AIDS is only a disease, and one which can be prevented. As yet, however, fatherhood and AIDS has not been widely discussed.

Sex and marriage

Listening to Ivorians, it appears that sexual habits have changed radically in the last 50 years. In the past there were strong taboos against sex before marriage, and a woman who became pregnant was the source of shame for herself and her parents. Now it is common for men and women to have sexual experience at an early age, and few unmarried mothers are rejected by their parents.

The first study of sexual behaviour in the Ivory Coast, involving 3,001 respondents across the country in 1989, showed that more than one in four men and almost one in five women were sexually active by the time they reached 14; by the age of 16, more than half of men and women were sexually active. In urban areas 60 percent of men claimed to be celibate or faithful to their sexual partners over the previous 12 months (although polygamy is illegal, many men have more than one regular partner); 40 percent of men had had at least one casual partner and one in every 12 men had five or more casual partners. In comparison, 88 percent of women said they had been celibate or faithful, and none claimed to have five or more sexual partners [11].

Overall, young men are most likely to have casual partners. Casual relationships are admitted by almost half of all men under 20 and more than half of all men between 20 and 24, but by only one in seven women under 20 and one in eight women between 20 and 24. By the time they reach their forties, only one in six men say they have casual sex [12].

In the past, a young man's parents would find a bride for their son. When the marriage was agreed, the engagement would be confirmed at a public ceremony. If the couple were still young, it might be several years before the wife went to live with her husband. Today, even in conservative rural areas, few parents now find spouses for their children, not least because family bonds are weakening as children as young as 12 move to a town or city to attend secondary school. Many men and women live together without marrying, or marry only after several years of living together. These partnerships may not be permanent or exclusive. Women tend to leave partners with whom they are not happy to find another man; as a result, many women have children by different fathers. Men tend to have several partners at the same time, living with a 'wife' and supporting one or more *mère(s) de mon enfant* ('mother(s) of my child'). Sometimes a man negotiates with his first wife for another woman to live with them; she may agree, on condition she receives a gift such as a sewing machine, shoes and cash.

Gifts of God

"I consider a child as the gift of God. I will continue having babies until they are finished in my womb," declares 40-year-old Awa from Bondoukou, in the north-east. She and her husband, a labourer, have six children and a seventh is on the way. Today, however, smaller families are becoming the norm. "I have three children, which I think is enough for me. If I had more I wouldn't have the means of taking care of them," says Magloire, 45, a teacher at Danane in the west of the country. "We are no longer living in the time of our fathers. They lived off the land and there was not much pressure on them. Then a child was considered a fortune. Now it has become a burden ."

Children are important in Ivorian society. Childless middle-aged women are often regarded with suspicion and considered witches; men of the same age without children are often considered irresponsible. On average, women first become pregnant when they are 18 or 19 and have three or four children [13]. There are no statistics for the age at which men first become fathers. Women who become pregnant before marriage often try to hide the pregnancy, but such a secret cannot be kept for ever. Whether through attendance at an ante-natal clinic or through the gossip of relatives or friends, a woman's family will hear of the situation. They are then likely to confront the father and insist that he (or his parents if he is too young to earn a living) provide for the child.

Births are still widely celebrated. Among the Baoulé, for

example, the infant's first hair is cut and mixed with leaves and palm wine, then given to the parents to drink (or to the mother and one of her brothers, if the father is not present). Then the party begins. Children are offered presents and a white ram may be killed and eaten.

Paternity

In Ivorian society the father is responsible for food, shelter and education. Among the Akan group, however, the children 'belong' to their mother's brother or brothers, who may contribute to their upbringing, sometimes taking all responsibility if the father is unable to do so. Although the law says that spouses and children are the primary inheritors, Akan children tend to inherit from their uncles, not their fathers. It is often said that Akan girls are better looked after than boys because it is their children who inherit the family's wealth.

Men with little education who live in fertile zones where land is available tend to have children at an early age. When he is about 20 years old, a young man often obtains the family's blessing to marry and is given his own home together with land or part of the family business to provide him and his children with an income. Rural men without land must migrate to fertile zones, where they work under contract and generally do not marry until they have saved enough money to support a family.

In urban areas most men also aim to save money before settling down, although if a man has not found a wife by the time he is 30 it is assumed to be a question of his reliability rather than his money. Men who are graduates tend to calculate everything. They meet their future wife at university and marry only when both have completed their studies, including time spent abroad. Relatives are informed of the couple's decision long before the wedding day. Children come only after the marriage, and there are unlikely to be more than three or four. Graduate men with girlfriends ensure that they do not become pregnant. Dr Youdjé Gnonsoa-Ateby of Population Services International points out that among wealthier Ivorians it is men who are concerned with the size and spacing of their families; in the poorer strata of society men used to take little part in family planning decisions, but are now beginning to take an interest.

The world comes to an end

Until recently many men hesitated about taking an HIV test unless they were very sick. Nowadays, as a result of widespread prevention campaigns, more and more men without symptoms take the test in confidential centres, particularly if they are in a serious long-term relationship. The incidence of HIV among men reaches its peak between the ages of 30 and 40, when most will already be fathers.

Young men's reaction to the news that they are HIV-positive is often very negative. Four months after receiving his diagnosis, Laurent, a young man in his twenties, continues to disbelieve it. "I can get to sleep every night only after praying for a long time. I think the test is wrong and want to do it again." Believing that their world has come to an end, some think about suicide – a few do kill themselves – and others abandon their work, even if they are not ill. In this confusion some stop having sexual relations, in the hope that a solution to their problem will be found. Dr Marc Aguirre, of the Centre d'Assistance Socio-Médicale (Centre for Social Medical Assistance) in Treichville, Abidjan, which works with lower-income men and women with HIV, says, "In general men seem to deny they are seropositive, and we have had to work hard on counselling." For a few men, learning that they have the virus has been an opportunity to take charge of their lives. Some become active in associations of people living with HIV.

To tell or not to tell

Many men who learn they have HIV do not inform their partners. Aguirre believes that this is true of the majority of his patients. "This is less because they are afraid of losing their partners than because of the stigma, the belief that they have lost a certain amount of dignity." As a result many women who are pregnant or have newborn children learn of their husband's seropositivity only from the death certificate. (Aguirre points out that many women also fail to inform their husbands, because they do not want to lose support. "The women who come here are very poor. They do not have a voice. They are economically dependent on one or two people.")

Thomas, a 40-year-old from Abidjan, says, "My wife reacted so badly when I tried to remind her that a man could be HIV-positive that I preferred not to talk about it to her any more. Since then we've had relations with a condom. More and more she wants to have a child and I am afraid of what might follow since, despite all my efforts, I haven't managed to convince her to take the HIV test." In contrast, perhaps because he was a father already, the family of François, a 50-year-old farmer, accepted the situation well. Several months after telling his wife that he was HIV-positive, he informed his children at a family reunion and lived the rest of his life at peace.

Sometimes the parents of a young man who is ill, whatever the disease, arrange a quick marriage to ensure that he fathers a child. In such a situation the young woman may not be aware of her husband's illness; indeed, the man may not have told the parents that he has HIV. This writer is aware of at least one such case, where a man died of AIDS leaving a young wife and child ignorant of the cause of his death and thus of the possibility that they had contracted the virus.

A sense of family

Sometimes men and their partners are tested when their baby falls ill and it is clear that the child has AIDS. In this situation some fathers do not accept that they may have brought the virus into the family, and it can be several months before they accept that they too may have HIV. In other cases the parents are concerned less with apportioning responsibility than with trying to resolve the problem of how to ensure their own survival and that of the child. The latter often requires considerable expenditure and several visits to hospital, often disrupting the family's everyday affairs.

Although not everyone agrees, fathers today seem closer to their children than their own fathers were, particularly among the middle class, although it is still women who spend most time with the children. There has been no in-depth study to discover whether men are more fatalistic and accept the illness and death of their children more easily than do women. It is this writer's opinion that men are indeed affected by a child's illness and are as upset as the mother on a child's death.

In one study of lower-income people with HIV in Abidjan, however, women appeared more likely than men to be concerned about the well-being of their children [14]. Marc Aguirre comments: "Women have a broader perspective: 'What does this [diagnosis] mean for me, my child, my family in general?'" Men, he goes on, tend to be more self-centred: "'What does this mean for me, my job, my place in the community?'"

Nevertheless, Aguirre believes that "the majority of men do still have a sense of family. They have children; they realise this will have repercussions on the family." Antoine, for example, a 42-year-old salesman with a wife and two adolescent daughters, wishes there was an insurance plan to guarantee payment of his children's school fees until they reach 21 [15]. However, according to the Abidjan study one of the factors which restricts the ability of lower-income men with HIV to contribute to their children's welfare is that they tend to receive less support from their extended families and others than do women in the same situation.

"To mark my time"

Men who are aware they are HIV-positive but who do not yet have children are faced with a difficult decision. Laurent Vidal, an AIDS expert, believes that most men and women with HIV find it difficult to agree not to have children. Alain Manouan of the National AIDS Programme, speaking about lower-income parents, agrees. He says that people believe that there is a one in two chance that the child will be seronegative (in contrast to the true figure, which is three in four): "So they say to themselves, 'Why not go ahead? I want a child and if the child is born HIV-positive, I'll do what I can so that it can live.'"

It has been suggested that women find it easier to accept the use of condoms, but in the experience of Robert Bouabi of the rural-based counselling organisation Village Virus they are more accepted by young men than young women in the same situation. "I suggested using a condom to a 19-year-old girl with HIV. She absolutely refused, saying she had to have a child."

Nevertheless, men with HIV who have not yet become fathers want children. Before he knew he had the virus, Marcel Bolou, a student and member of Le Club des Amis (The Friends' Club), an organisation for men and women living with HIV, says he wanted four children, two of each sex. Now he will be content with one child "to mark my time on this earth". However, even though he knows there is only a one in four chance of mother-child transmission, he is afraid of passing the virus to a future child and causing the infant to suffer. Bolou would prefer to meet a woman who is HIV-positive, but "if I meet a woman who is seronegative and she accepts my condition, then perhaps we can have a relationship." In that case they will take precautions to try and protect her from contracting the virus, and if she does so, zidovudine may reduce the likelihood of the child also contracting it.

Désiré Ndah Koua, also of Le Club des Amis, is in a relationship with a woman who is HIV-negative. Although Ndah already has seven children by other mothers and would be happy not to become a father again, his partner wants to have his child. "We take care," he says. "We use a condom except when she has her fertile days, and she has the system which tells her which days these are."

Children with HIV, children who are orphaned

As indicated above, over 15,000 of the 700,000 children born each year in the Ivory Coast are likely to be HIV-positive. A further 400,000 children have lost one or both parents to the disease since the start of the epidemic, a number expected to double by 2005 [16]. AIDS aside, the loss of a parent for any reason causes great pain for children, and the younger they are, the greater the sense of loss. When the father works and pays for the family expenses, the wife takes over after his death. When it is the mother who dies, the situation is more difficult. With the death of Marie, for example, a street-vendor from the Treichville district of Abidjan, her family fell apart. The older children disappeared and the younger ones are being looked after by different families.

Various institutions work with the extended families of children orphaned by the epidemic to ease their suffering. In some cases financial and material support is offered for their upkeep and education. "We prefer to let the children stay with family members, so they can grow up and maintain the extended family system," says Sister Dr Lucie Maule, a nun at the Sister Dorothe Education and Health Centre in Alepe.

"We give them support through outreach programmes and monitor their growth and development. This way we think we are doing them more good than by confining them in orphanages." However, the Centre does also operate an orphanage for abandoned children.

The Centre offers small amounts of money to HIV-positive mothers, enabling them to engage in petty trading, the profits from which are used to look after their dependants. "The approach is working very well, enabling hard working beneficiaries to double what we give them in a comparatively short period," says project coordinator Hubert Ahouassa.

Community support

With the arrival of AIDS many associations have been created – or have extended their activities – to bring information to communities in even the smallest provinces. NGOs and associations of people living with HIV/AIDS include Lumière Action, Le Club des Amis, GAP+PS (Group to Help People Living with HIV/AIDS and Social Promotion, of which this writer is president), Virus Village and, most recently, Amepouh ('We will win' in the Guéré language), which brings together women with HIV.

There is often a lively debate within the associations of people living with HIV over whether a man or woman with the virus should have children. People have been criticised for conceiving a child – by people who themselves later decide to become a parent. These and other organisations offer counselling for potential parents with HIV, but there is still a long way to go before every man with the virus clearly understands the implications of transmission and the options for conception and contraception that are open to him.

Of perhaps more immediate concern is the fact that although many organisations work with HIV-positive mothers, no programmes exist to help fathers with the virus look after their children.

The responsibilities of men

In the world of HIV/AIDS there are many references to mother-child transmission, but none to father-child transmission. Should this change? Can more be done to teach HIV-positive men the risks of passing the virus to their children? Should the risk of father-child transmission play a prominent role in future prevention campaigns? Dr Alain Manouan of the National AIDS Programme says, "That depends on the public. If you address people with some education, they will understand that father-child transmission passes through the mother. If you speak to people with little education, it could lead to confusion."

Men have responsibilities towards their children, whether or not they are HIV-positive. That includes recognising their paternity, working to ensure that they have enough to eat each day, and also ensuring that they have an education and/or skills to allow them to feed themselves once they become adults. In other words, they must prepare for their children's future, especially if the children may become orphans. None of this is possible if fathers with HIV do not have the courage and honesty to inform their partners of their infection.

O MY BROTHERS, DRIVERS AND HELPERS!

INTRODUCTION

If there is any nation where encouraging men to change their sexual behaviour can have an immediate impact on the HIV/AIDS epidemic, it is Bangladesh. One of the poorest countries on the planet, it has high rates of illiteracy and sexually transmitted disease, although – surprisingly – not of HIV. Most men and women, particularly in the large rural population, adhere to sexual roles that allow wives little or no control over their sexual lives. Nevertheless, considerable progress has been made in the nearly 30 years since independence; nationwide family planning and microcredit programmes as well as immunisation against childhood diseases have begun a process of widespread social change, the full impact of which is still unclear.

At first glance it might seem that Bangladesh's experience in family planning would allow it to implement an effective nationwide HIV/AIDS prevention programme quickly. However, unlike HIV prevention, family planning does not require men's knowledge or consent. New strategies must therefore be devised, and Mostafa Kamal Majumder highlights several innovative programmes in which non-governmental organisations are bringing information about HIV/AIDS to men who are most at risk.

In the programmes described here, the organisers and their target audience often have very different goals. The Aricha Ghat health and recreation centre, for example, was opened specifically to inform men about HIV/AIDS, but the truck drivers and helpers who use it see it primarily as a place where they can wash and relax while waiting for the ferry. Establishing these programmes has been a learning process for the educators as much as for the target audience. As Majumder reports, one organisation took pains to gain the trust of its target audience through entertainment such as drama and cricket and through group counselling sessions, but it took time to recognise that the men of the village, who were their most important target, were more easily reached in the nearby town, where they worked in the docks and slept in dormitories.

It is too early to learn which programmes are effective in changing men's behaviour, but these are early days and both the men at risk and the men and women who work with them have much to learn.

EDUCATING MEN ABOUT HIV/AIDS IN BANGLADESH

by Mostafa Kamal Majumder

By early 1998 sporadic nationwide testing had identified only 102 people with HIV in a total population of over 125 million. This apparently low prevalence, particularly given the high rates of other sexually transmitted infections (STIs, also known as STDs) in Bangladesh, is an "epidemiological mystery", according to Professor M Nazrul Islam of the Bangladesh AIDS Prevention and Control Programme.

Among the people discovered to be HIV-positive, men outnumber women by more than five to one. Many if not most of the men probably contracted the virus while working abroad – over two million Bangladeshis (all but 12,000 of whom are men) are migrant workers in the Gulf States, Malaysia and other Asian countries. However, none of the women known to have HIV, who include housewives and sex workers, have ever left the country. This confirmation that indigenous transmission has already occurred has led

UNAIDS to estimate that 20,000 Bangladeshis may have contracted the virus.

Men and women

Bangladesh is a conservative, Muslim country where pre-marital and extramarital sex is not only frowned upon but illegal. To prevent them from coming into contact with the opposite sex, women are traditionally forbidden to socialise with men outside their family. Many parents still select spouses for their sons and daughters. While men are permitted more than one wife (although few exercise this option), women must remain faithful to their only husband.

Officially, therefore, men and women have sex only within marriage. In reality sexual behaviour is more complex. Widespread sexually transmitted disease – between one in 50 and one in 100 pregnant women suffer from syphilis or gonorrhoea – provides evidence of extensive extramarital activity. Prostitution is illegal but commercial sex workers are licensed, and brothel complexes with up to 1,000 working women can be found in or near large cities. On average, each woman serves five clients a day, from businessmen to students, truck drivers to rickshaw pullers. Recent studies show a significant number of men have sex with other men.

Infidelity by men is tolerated for a number of reasons, including the commonly held perception that they have a greater need for sex. Dr Hasan Mahmood, director of the government's STD Project, suggests that both men and women are equally motivated to have intercourse but men are freer to express and fulfil their sexual desire. Paradoxically, Dr Hasan suggests, this offers women a temporary advantage. Since the experience that would be gained from pre-marital sex is theoretically forbidden, many young men are afraid of sex when they get married, while women appear to be less nervous in the same situation.

After marriage, however, the roles are reversed. Economic dependence and lack of security compel many women to tolerate their husband's demands for sex or extramarital relationships. "When wives feel no sex urge, they normally remain silent and inactive as the husband releases his body tension," says Dr Hasan. He believes that domestic violence is rare but the fear generated in such situations is "like sexual abuse or rape, against which women have no place to complain".

Men and men

Recent studies suggest that between one and three percent of Bangladeshi men occasionally or regularly have sex with other men, a figure that represents between 300,000 and 900,000 men. Dr Suman Lahiry of the Association for Health and Social Development (AHSD) claims that men who have sex with men can be found in all sections of society. Some have been educated in Europe or North America and identify as gay, while many more are married to women and consider themselves heterosexual.

Because the law criminalises and marginalises men who have sex with men, says Lahiry, there is no gay culture as known in Western countries, institutions such as male brothels do not exist and male sex workers are not registered. The commonest way for men to contact each other is in parks in the evening, where there are informal networks of men who sell and buy sex. Slang, incomprehensible to the general population, is used to identify potential partners and different sex acts. Not every sexual act is accompanied by exchange of money, although some researchers believe that most sex between men in Bangladesh has a financial component.

Abul, a sex worker who can often be found in Ramna and Osmany parks in the capital, Dhaka, says that most male sex workers' clients are Bangladeshis, although he and others sometimes find foreign clients through staff working in expensive hotels. Two other sex workers in the parks questioned for this report have some knowledge about sexually transmitted diseases and have taken medicines to cure ailments from time to time, but they are not fully aware of the means by which HIV is transmitted. They continue to have penetrative sex, although they wash their anus every night with antiseptic liquids in the belief that this will protect them.

Some male sex workers are eunuchs (*hijras*), who are usually castrated at a young age by older *hijras*. *Hijras* and some men dress as women, take hormone pills to enlarge their beasts and refer to themselves and each other as 'she'. These hormones are almost always taken without medical supervision and can lead to significant medical problems such as cancer.

Not all sex between men is consensual. Male rape occurs at places such as truck stands, jetties and even in Dhaka parks. Restaurant boys and unregistered 'coolies' (labourers) at railway stations face sexual abuse by their employers and older workers. Overall, however, male rape is believed to be rare.

Family planning

In the past sex was seldom discussed, but this began to change with the introduction of widespread family planning in the early 1980s. Nevertheless, there remains considerable ignorance of a range of sexual matters, including diseases such as AIDS. The most recent demographic and health survey (1996-97) indicated that no more than three in every 10 men and two in every 10 women had heard about AIDS, knew how it was spread and how to avoid contracting HIV. Despite this widespread ignorance, however, many people are hopeful that the successful implementation of other health programmes means a serious epidemic can be avoided. The country has a high rate of child immunisation, and the incidence of childhood diarrhoea, responsible for 150,000 deaths each year, appears to be falling.

The country's spectacular success in reducing the population growth rate seems to have relevance to the anti-AIDS drive. Contraceptive use by married women increased from one in 10 to five in 10 between 1975 and 1996, and fertility fell from 6.3 to 3.27 children in the same period. A number of factors were responsible for this success, including strong political commitment, a nationwide media campaign and inclusion of the subject in school and college curricula, increased empowerment of women, combining maternal and child health care with family planning services and better rates of child survival.

Perhaps the most important factor, according to Dr Ahmed Al Sabir of the government's National Institute of Population Research and Training (NIPORT), was the employment of 23,000 women Family Welfare Assistants (FWAs) to take family planning messages to married women across the country. FWAs have easy access to mothers and supply contraceptives free of charge. Their job itself acts as a role model and encourages women to work outside the family home. A parallel development – the creation of income-generating activities for women by non-governmental organisations (NGOs) – has enabled more mothers to contribute to the family income and have a greater say in decisions, such as the preferred number of children.

Initially, the greatest obstacle to the family planning programme was the attitude of imams, who instruct the faithful and lead prayers in mosques. Births and deaths were previously viewed as dictates of God; some mullahs (experts in Islamic law) decried family planning and refused to lead funeral prayers for those who had undergone vasectomy and tubectomy. Once religious leaders were persuaded of the need, however, they began to inform their congregations about ways of keeping family size manageable, such as delayed marriage, restraint and premature withdrawal. Now imams frequently answer questions from radio listeners on the use of family planning methods in the light of Islam.

Reaching men

Although the family planning programme has been successful in its approach to certain aspects of sexuality, Subrata Kumar Bhadra of NIPORT warns that not all the same techniques can be applied directly to HIV/AIDS prevention. Family planning is directed at married women, and very few men and relatively few teenagers are addressed. Furthermore, the emphasis has been on female methods of contraception, with only four percent of married couples relying on condoms to prevent pregnancy. Nevertheless, although programmes to prevent the spread of HIV/AIDS are still at a formative phase, some have started giving encouraging results and information.

"Men are a decisive group in respect of sex," says Professor Islam of the AIDS Prevention and Control Programme. They have much greater freedom than women, are sexually more active and, because they often have more than one partner, are critical in disseminating the virus. Prevention programmes "should not only diagnose and treat the STDs of people belonging to their target groups, but also create in them self-esteem." Thus programmes deal with the mechanics of HIV transmission and, where circumstances allow, encourage men to understand how male norms and ego make them, their wives and offspring vulnerable to the disease.

Because they are socially and economically mobile, men are harder to contact than women. NGOs have begun to work with groups of men who are away from their families for long periods, during which they often seek extramarital sex. These include truck drivers and their helpers, emigrant workers, rickshaw pullers, slum-dwellers, residents of mess homes (dormitories for men who cannot bring their families to town), seafarers and dockworkers as well as intravenous drug users (an estimated 200,000 people, mostly men) and men who have sex with men.

While most programmes are based in and around Dhaka, activities also take place in other towns and cities, such as the seaport of Chittagong. Most programmes begin with an assessment of the needs of the target groups – the knowledge they have and the knowledge they need to protect themselves and their partners from sexually transmitted infections, including HIV. In theory, the success or failure of the programmes is measured by such indicators as whether the prevalence of infections and the use of condoms rises or falls among the members of the target groups, but there have been no such surveys so far.

"O my brothers, drivers and helpers!"

There are estimated to be over 300,000 truck drivers and their helpers in Bangladesh, who are at high risk of contracting HIV because of their frequent absences from home and their sexual contacts with prostitutes and, in some cases, with each other. Many of these drivers pass through Aricha Ghat, where about 2,000 trucks and over 1,000 other vehicles are ferried daily between eastern and western Bangladesh across the Jamuna (Brahmaputra) river. During the hours, sometimes days, that truck drivers and helpers queue at the Ghat, many visit brothels.

The lack of a place for rest and recreation, of clean toilets and places to wash led the non-government organisation CEDAR (Concern for Environmental Development and Research) to open a health and recreation centre in a two-storey tin shed near the ferry in January 1996. The centre has since become popular among drivers and their helpers, who learn about it from Sadeque, a dancer-cum-folk singer employed by CEDAR. Crowds gather as Sadeque dances and sings and he and other outreach workers distribute brochures on the centre's activities.

O my brothers, drivers and helpers!
A disease has broken out, this disease has no cure!

O my brothers, drivers and helpers!
They call it AIDS, I tell you all.

O my brothers, drivers and helpers!
A disease has broken out, this disease has no cure!

Always remember – if the blood of one enters another!

O my brothers, drivers and helpers!
A disease has broken out, this disease has no cure!

Anyone can use the centre, but to create a sense of belonging drivers and helpers are encouraged to take out membership at a cost of Taka 20 (US$0.50) and Taka 10 (US$0.25) respectively. By the end of 1997 over 1,100 drivers and helpers had joined, together with ferry terminal workers, who also live away from home for long periods. There are clean latrines and bathing places, and recreation facilities include *carom* (a game similar to billiards or pool), cards, chess, newspapers, radio and television. The centre shows films on STI/AIDS awareness, offers free examinations by a doctor and free medicines, and makes condoms available in the toilets and on demand.

According to Mahbooba Akhter Kabita of HASAB (HIV/AIDS STD Activities in Bangladesh), which supports the centre, "The drivers and helpers place greater emphasis on sanitation facilities and entertainment than on STD services." However, this does not mean that the centre is failing in its primary goal of helping prevent the transmission of disease. Initial studies show that eight out of every 10 drivers and helpers had an infection. Before the centre opened, the shame associated with these diseases prevented many drivers from seeking help, but now they are able to talk freely to the CEDAR staff and receive treatment. Abu Sayeed, a health educator at the centre, says that rising demand for condoms reflects increased awareness about risky sexual behaviour among truck drivers and their helpers. Every day 25 to 30 men visit the centre for condoms, many of them returning with their colleagues on subsequent trips.

Fish processors

Thousands of men and women are employed in 27 shrimp processing factories in Char Rupsha, 335 kilometres south-west of Dhaka. Most come from the surrounding districts of Faridpur, Madaripur and Satkhira, and almost all live in slums away from their families, moving from one factory to another for work. During the busy season workers can earn Taka 1,500 (US$39) a month. Hours are not fixed; when there is an adequate supply of fish, work continues day and night.

Men and women live separately, the men in mess houses in which 10 to 15 people share a room. Many of the women are married with children but have been deserted by their husbands. As earnings from the fish processing factories are low, many female workers sell sex and sometimes are compelled to have sex with their employers.

The youth-oriented NGO Jagrata Juba Sangha (JJS), with financial support from HASAB, provides information on HIV/AIDS to women and men, approaching them at their mess homes and meeting them two to three times a month. JJS has also persuaded some factory owners and managers to allow them to hold discussions on the premises. The workers are under no obligation to attend the lectures or to interact with the health educators during group discussions. Workers can also see a doctor and be treated for sexually transmitted infections at the JJS centre, where they can buy condoms at nominal prices.

Discussions follow a pattern used by other groups supported by HASAB. They usually begin with everyday matters. "This gives us two advantages," explains Mahbooba

Akhtar Kabita. "First it enables the educator to learn about the practices of group members, and how these practices make them vulnerable to STDs. He can then disseminate information in keeping with the information that comes through discussion."

When rapport has been established, members of target groups, who are mostly unmarried young men, ask questions about topics that concern them. The men may previously have talked to traditional healers who play their trade in marketplaces, often giving erroneous sexual advice. Typical subjects at the JJS discussions include masturbation and how to increase 'sex power'. The aim of the educator is not to make individuals feel guilty, but to respect whatever acts they may have engaged in. This encourages members of the target group to become more open about discussing their behaviour in detail.

A gradual approach

JJS's work is not easy. According to Hasina Begum who works with the organisation, workers are teased by some young people who call them "healers of penis-related diseases". They have also been abused by women for initiating discussion of sex. The women were angry at the open discussion of 'secret matters', which they feared made them appear to be sinners, and they thought that the health educators had evil motives. A.T.M. Zakir Hossain, executive director of JJS, says people used to ask angrily if they were out to lure young people into committing sin. "Some of our workers came back and wept as they narrated the experience of resistance. We changed our approach and tried to understand the needs of the people at risk and tried to help them by sinking tube-wells for safe drinking water and by extending microcredit. We talked to influential people, owners of fish processing factories and owners of slums, and explained to them the danger of the spread of AIDS. We gradually started talking about HIV/AIDS and sex."

In time attitudes change. Thanks to the programme Mashiur Rahman, 28, knows that people can contract AIDS through "illegal mixing" (sex), used syringe needles and used razor blades at barbers' shops. He says, "There is no cure for AIDS. However, if we lead decent lives and protect ourselves from the virus we will not get the disease." He points out that most male fish processing workers try to satisfy their sexual urge by going to "forbidden places" (brothels) at night. "Maybe those who are aware of the dangers of unprotected sex use condoms." He believes, however, that both men and women complain they do not get full sexual satisfaction when condoms are used. Project manager Fatima Aktar is not disappointed by his reaction. "There is substance in the statement," Aktar comments, but adds that, "Condom promotion is still useful because those who do the act 'illegally' do not expect full satisfaction."

Deedarul Alam, 28, who worked at the Jahanabad Fish Processing plant, says that he has learned much from attending JJS lectures and group discussions. Sheikh Ishtiaque, 23, had heard about AIDS, "which is a dreadful disease", before coming to Char Rupsha but he did not know its details. "After listening to the lectures, I now know how the disease spreads," he says, and understands that syphilis and gonorrhoea are spread in the same way.

Dock labourers

Demand for condoms has increased in the village of Pailatala, about 400 kilometres south-west of Dhaka, where 435 dock labourers' families are gradually becoming aware of the dangers of unsafe sex. In the past condoms used to be distributed by family planning workers in the villages, and were available at chemists in the nearby town of Morrelganj. Now they are available at grocery shops in the villages, according to Nasiruddin Talukdar, executive director of the Community Development Centre (CDC), which has introduced an HIV/AIDS prevention programme there.

The docks are in Mongla, a town 20 kilometres away that can be reached from the village only by boat; some men travel regularly from the village, while others sleep in dormitories in the town. Dockworkers may stay away from their homes for weeks and are a high-risk group for contracting HIV because nearly 75 percent of them have STDs, says Nasiruddin. Some workers say that after 10 days or more away from their families their "blood heats up" and they need sex.

Initially the response to CDC's programme was poor, although the organisation had already established itself as a self-sustaining microcredit organisation that was benefiting about 4,000 families in the locality. Talukdar describes how his team won over the doubters. "First we enquired about their welfare. Then we slowly initiated discussion on sex, terming it a part of life, and then discussed STDs. As we got closer to them we sought to get to know their personal problems, which they had previously hidden. They became so intimate with us that they told us things they did not even share with their friends. We told them that there was another disease that was also contracted through sex but was incurable."

In their first year of work CDC activists promoted sports and games for adolescents, to fill their spare time. In 1997 the World AIDS Day programme at Morrelganj included a drama with messages on HIV/AIDS and a cricket tournament, as well as rallies and discussions in which important local people took part.

Despite these activities CDC realised that visits to Pailatala and group were inadequate for the task. Dockworkers are an important target, but when CDC workers were holding counselling sessions in dockworkers' villages, most of the workers were in Mongla. CDC, therefore, began discussion groups with dockworkers in Mongla, and the frequency of visit to brothels by dockworkers appears to be coming down.

Hidden men

One of the toughest challenges for AIDS prevention workers is reaching men who have sex with men. Suman Lahiry of the Association for Health and Social Development insists that unless adequate prevention programmes are targeted at this group, the national AIDS programme will fail, as without adequate information men who have sex with men run a high risk of contracting HIV and passing the virus to their women partners.

Men who contract a disease from sex with another man may go to one of the few STD clinics, but the surgeries are often crowded and doctors avoid discussing all aspects of the illnesses with patients. In particular, both doctor and patient may be prevented by *lajja* (shame) from discussing sex between men and problems related to anal sex. In such circumstances doctors may refer patients to clinics specialising in haemorrhoids or, because of the stigma attached to anal sex, discuss the subject in demeaning and abusive terms instead of offering medical treatment.

Male sex workers, because they have frequent sex, face even greater problems. Because most doctors refuse to treat them, they often rely on *kaviraj* (traditional healers), who are not always reliable and who have been found selling AIDS Malam (a lotion that is claimed to be an AIDS cure). According to one expert, traditional healers may have a role in discussing and raising awareness of sexually transmitted diseases, but they need training and motivation in order to do so.

Strong condoms reduce the risk of HIV transmission during sex between men. However, because condoms available for family planning are not generally approved for anal sex, some male sex workers do not use them. Instead they use oily lubricants which do not protect against HIV and which some experts consider carcinogenic.

Programmes for men who have sex with men are recent.

It will be an uphill task to reach many in the target group, particularly those who allege that they are subject to abuse and physical harassment by law enforcement agencies, who exploit them both in terms of money and sex. Indeed, when first approached by researchers many of the men were afraid that the researchers would register them with police; rapport had to be built up before these fears were allayed. While this report was being written, regular group discussions had not yet begun.

Cause for optimism?

These examples give some idea of the AIDS prevention programmes being developed in Bangladesh by NGOs. In 1993 a network of NGOs working in STD/AIDS was established with 24 members. Four years later that number had risen to 200, about 50 of which have long-term programmes with high-risk groups such as migrant workers.

Other programmes targeted at men include awareness campaigns in university dormitories and higher secondary-level colleges. Some teachers originally protested against the use of messages about condoms, but in most cases NGOs have managed to design messages that are acceptable to both staff and students. Limited programmes have also started for intravenous drug users.

According to Dr Nasir Uddin, chairperson of the STD/AIDS network, some of the original messages spread by network members through posters and leaflets were misleading, but this is no longer the case. At the moment it is difficult to assess whether NGO activities have led to behavioural change, but there has been a noticeable increase in the sale of condoms and Uddin is optimistic that further results will be visible by 2000.

The message is spreading

Despite the rapid rise in the number of HIV/AIDS prevention programmes, they are still far from meeting the country's needs. The scale of the problem can be seen in the fact that it is estimated that half a million rickshaw pullers work in Dhaka alone. And while many clients of sex workers, seen as a key group, are targeted through programmes for groups of workers such as truck drivers and dockers, others such as businessmen, students and white collar workers slip through the net.

Furthermore, many day-to-day problems face existing programmes. As described above, people are often hostile to HIV/AIDS workers at the first meeting. Sometimes the response is physical. Sadeque, who works with CEDAR, was once slapped by a truck driver when he talked about sex. But when the confidence of the target group is gained, the work is much easier. "People do not cooperate if confidentiality is not assured," says Professor Nazrul. NGO workers also find that offering a range of services, such as treatment of STDs and recreation facilities, generates a better response.

The AIDS Prevention and Control Programme in Bangladesh has taken a big step forward in recent years. The adoption of the National AIDS Policy and the five-year strategic plan theoretically place the country years ahead of its neighbours. A wide range of groups at risk are now specifically targeted and the message is spreading. As a result of these activities a non-permissive, conservative society has begun to tolerate open discussion of sex. Free distribution and increased sales of condoms and an indication that STD rates in some groups may have begun to fall suggest that men have indeed begun to change their behaviour. If these activities are consolidated and strengthened, the prevalence of HIV in Bangladesh may remain low.

Notes

Men, Sex and HIV

1. 'Sexual behaviour in developing countries: implications for HIV control', M Caraël et al, *AIDS*, 1995, vol 9, no 10, pp1171–1175
2. *Primera Encuesta Nacional Sobre SIDA*, Johnny Madrigal & Jacobo Schifter, Asociación Demográfica Costarricense, San José, 1990
3. *Sexual Behaviour in Britain*, Kaye Wellings et al, Penguin, London, 1994, pp95–96
4. Damien Rwegera, quoted in *HIV and the Challenges Facing Men*, Kathryn Carovano, Issues Paper 15, HIV and Development Programme, UNDP, New York, 1995
5. Report by AIDS prevention worker in Rajasthan, *Naz Ki Pukaar*, no 5, 1994
6. According to the definition used here, sex workers comprise only part of a core group, since their vulnerability to the virus depends on interaction with their clients, who form the other part.
7. Rates of HIV infection or frequency of sexual intercourse are not necessarily uniform in a core group; for example, sex workers often have more frequent sex and higher rates of infection than their clients.
8. 'Sexual behaviour in India with risk of HIV/AIDS transmission', Moni Nag, *Health Transition Review*, supplement to vol 5, 1995, p297
9. 'Male knowledge of and attitudes and practices towards *AIDS*', D Adamchak et al, AIDS, 1990, vol 4, p245
10. *Sexual Ecology: AIDS and the destiny of gay men*, Gabriel Rotello, Dutton, New York, 1997, p61
11. A different analysis comes to the same conclusion. In a theoretical community in which 250 married men and 50 unpartnered women have unprotected sex with more than one partner and all other adults in the community either abstain from sex or are faithful to their partners, not only the 300 men and women but also the faithful wives of the 250 men are liable to contract HIV. Ultimately,

therefore, 250 men and 300 women (50 unpartnered women and 250 wives) may become HIV-positive and for five out of every six women with the virus, the only risk factor will have been intercourse with their long-term partners.

12. *AIDS in the World II*, eds Jonathan M Mann & Daniel J. M. Tarantola, Oxford University Press, 1996, p465

13. Figures extrapolated from 'Sexual transmission of HIV', Rachel A Royce et al, *New England Journal of Medicine*, 10 April 1997, pp1072–1078

14. 2.3 times riskier than vaginal intercourse, according to 'Male-to-female transmission of Human Immunodeficiency Virus', Nancy Padian et al, *Journal of the American Medical Association*, 14 August 1987, vol 258, no 6, pp788–790; a risk of between one in 30 and one in 200 penetrative acts, according to *Confronting AIDS: Public Priorities in a Global Epidemic*, World Bank/Oxford University Press, 1997, p59

15. *Debonair*, date not known, reproduced in *Sexuality and Sexual Behaviour in India*, Naz Foundation, London, no date

16. 'HIV prevention among Zambian adolescents', Douglas A Feldman et al, *Social Sciences Medicine*, 1997, vol 44, no 4, pp455–468

17. POPLINE abstract of *Lack of evidence for transmission of human immunodeficiency virus through vaginal intercourse*, S Brody, *Archives of Sexual Behaviour*, August 1995, 24 (4), pp383–93

18. *On the Margins*, Neil McKenna, Panos/Norwegian Red Cross, London, 1996

19. 1995 figure; see 'Global epidemiology of sexually transmitted diseases', Antonio C Gerbase et al, *Sexually Transmitted Diseases*, supplement to *The Lancet*, June 1998

20. Chancroid, syphilis and herpes are associated with a 1.5– to sevenfold increase in risk of infection; gonorrhoea, chlamydia and trichomonas infection with a 60 to 340 percent increase; statistics from 'Sexual transmission of HIV', op cit [note 13].

21. The procedure of genital mutilation may also lead to transmission of HIV and other diseases if the equipment is used on more than one person and is not sterilised between uses.

22. See various references on several African countries quoted in 'Local voices: what some Harare men say about preparation for sex', Sunanda Ray et al, *Reproductive Health Matters*, May 1996, 7, pp34–45; see also: 'Does intravaginal preparation use increase STD and HIV transmission in Zimbabwe?', Janneke Van de Wijgert, Abstract 23371, Conference Record, 12th World AIDS Conference, Geneva, 1998

23. Viral load is also high when an indidividual is seriously ill with AIDS, but the desire for sex is likely to be much less at that time.

24. 'Sexual transmission of HIV', op cit [note 13]

25. 'A model-based estimate of HIV infectivity via needle sharing', Edward H Kaplan & Robert Heimer, *Journal of Acquired Immune Deficiency Syndromes*, 1992, vol 5, pp1116–1118

26. In line with those who see female circumcision as genital mutilation, some commentators, while recognising that the risks involved are generally less serious, also identify male circumcision as genital mutilation.

27. 'Sexual transmission of HIV', op cit [note 13]; for a discussion of the issue, see 'The East Africa AIDS epidemic and the absence of male circumcision: what is the link?', two papers with same title (authors: T.E. Mertens & M Carael; S Moses et al), *Health Transition Review*, April 1995, 5 (1), pp100–108

28. 'Differential growth of HIV-1 subtypes in Langerhans' Cells; relation to transmission route', Luis E Soto-Ramirez et al, *Abstracts of the XI International Conference on AIDS*, TuA370, Vancouver, 1996

29. 'HIV-1 subtype RNA levels in semen of HIV-1 infected Thai men does not explain the apparent preference for subtype E being more readily transmitted sexually than subtype-B-Thai', Robert W Coombs et al, Abstract 23395, 12th World AIDS Conference, Geneva, 1998

30. For further discussion, see: 'How many HIV infections cross the bisexual bridge? An estimate from the United States', James G Kahn et al, *AIDS*, 1997, vol 11, pp1031–1037

31. *Sexual Ecology*, op cit [note 10] pp38–64

32. 'Heterosexual transmission of HIV in Haiti', Marie-Marcelle Deschamps et al, *Annals of Internal Medicine*, 1996, 125, pp324–330

33. 'Two million HIV infections prevented in Thailand: estimate of the impact of increased condom use', Noah Jamiel Robinson et al, *Abstracts of the XI International Conference on AIDS*, MoC904, Vancouver, 1996

34. 'Identifying condom users at risk for breakage and slippage: findings from three international sites', A Spruyt et al, *American Journal of Public Health*, 1998, 88 (2), pp239–44; 'Why do condoms break or slip off in use?', Juliet Richters et al, *International Journal of STD and AIDS*, 1995, 6, pp11–18

35. 'Violence, rape and sexual coercion: everyday love in a South African township', K Wood and R Jewkes, in *Men and Masculinity*, ed C Sweetman, Oxfam, 1997

36. For example, 'Female condom re-use: assessing structural integrity after multiple wash, dry and re-lubrication cycles', James McIntyre et al, Abstract 33124, 12th World AIDS Conference, Geneva, 1998

37. 'Experiences of 100 men who have sex with men using the female condom for anal sex', Daniel Wohlfeiler et al, Abstract 33133, 12th World AIDS Conference, Geneva, 1998

38. SEA-AIDS (internet) discussion, August 1998; see also 'Misunderstanding of 'safer sex' by heterosexually active adults', NS Wenger et al, *Public Health Reports*, September/October 1995, vol 110, no 5, pp618–621

39. For a more detailed analysis of HIV epidemiology, see *Confronting AIDS*, op cit [note 14]

40. 'HIV infection and sexually transmitted diseases', Mead Over and Peter Piot, paper published by Population, Health and Nutrition Division of the World Bank, Washington DC, 1991, quoted in *AIDS and the World*, eds Jonathan Mann et al, Harvard, 1992, p186

41. *Confronting AIDS*, op cit [note 14] p135

WHAT MAKES A MAN?

1. See *Sex on the Brain*, Deborah Blum, Viking, New York, 1997; and *How the Mind Works*, Steven Pinker, Norton, New York 1997

2. For example, presentation by Lynne Segal, Professor of Gender at Middlesex University, London, session D13 at 12th World AIDS Conference, Geneva, 1998

3. *HIV and the Challenges Facing Men*, Kathryn Carovano, Issues Paper 15, HIV and Development Programme, UNDP/Kumarian, New York, 1995, p4

4. Adapted from 'Under the blanket: bisexualities and AIDS in India', Shivananda Khan, in *Bisexualities and AIDS: International Perspectives*, ed Peter Aggleton, Taylor & Francis, London, 1996, p164

5. This practice appears to be dying in some cultures where it was once common; see *The Meanings of Macho: Being a Man in Mexico City*, Matthew C Gutmann, University of California, 1996; and 'Sexual cultures and sexual health: young people and their current discourse, practice and risks regarding sexuality in Lima, Peru', Carlos F Caceres, *Abstracts of the XI International Conference on AIDS*, ThD440, Vancouver, 1996

6. 'Thai views of sexuality and sexual behaviour', J Knodel et al, *Health Transition Review*, 1996, vol 6, pp179–201

7. 'Migrancy, masculine identities and AIDS: the psychosocial context of HIV transmission on the South African gold mines', C Campbell, *Social Sciences Medicine*, 1997, vol 45 no 2, pp273–281

8. 'Under the blanket', op cit [note 4] p168
9. *Sexual Ecology: AIDS and the destiny of gay men*, Gabriel Rotello, Dutton, New York, 1997, p203
10. Presentation by Lynne Segal, op cit [note 2]
11. 'Strengthening women's rights to protect themselves against sexual transmission of HIV: an educational programme in Zaire', Marie-Louise Ndala Musuamba, *Newsletter of the African Network on Ethics, Law and HIV*, December 1996, no 2, p4
12. 'Bisexuality and HIV/AIDS in Mexico', Ana Luisa Liguori et al, in *Bisexualities and AIDS*, op cit [note 4] pp76–98
13. According to Professor Dede Oetomo from Indonesia, some men believe that insertive oral intercourse with transvestites cleanses the penis, while Shivananda Khan of the Naz Foundation says South Asian men often consider sex with other men as less significant than with their wives.
14. 'Violence, rape and sexual coercion: everyday love in a South African township', K Wood and R Jewkes, in *Men and Masculinity*, ed C Sweetman, Oxfam, 1997
15. Statistics quoted in 'Consequences of sexual abuse of adolescents', Lindsay Stewart et al, *Reproductive Health Matters*, May 1996, no 7, pp129–134
16. 'Men, masculinities and the politics of development', Sarah C White, in *Men and Masculinity*, op cit [note 14]
17. 'Living with HIV/AIDS: a personal testimony', R Seruunkuma, *AIDS Health Promotion Exchange*, 1994, vol 3, p7, quoted in *Facing the Challenges of HIV/AIDS/STDs: A gender-based response*, Royal Tropical Institute (KIT) et al, Amsterdam, 1995, p14
18. 'Local voices: what some Harare men say about preparation for sex', Sunanda Ray et al, *Reproductive Health Matters*, May 1996, 7, pp34–45
19. Women also sexually and physically abuse children and men, but there is some controversy as to the extent to which this happens and little research has been undertaken into its frequency.
20. *Sexism and the War System*, B Reardon, Teachers College Press, New York, 1985, quoted in 'The origins and control of domestic violence against women', Soledad Larrain & Teresa Rodríguez, in *Gender, Women and Health in the Americas*, Pan American Health Organization, Washington DC, 1993
21. 'Self-esteem is essential', Patricia Burke, in *HIV and AIDS: The Global Inter-Connection*, ed Elizabeth Reid, UNDP/Kumarian, New York, 1995, pp157–165
22. *Sexual Ecology*, op cit [note 9] p139
23. 'Some cultural underpinnings of male sexual behaviour patterns in

Thailand', Mark Vanlandingham and Nancy Grandjean, in *Sexual Cultures and Migration in the Era of AIDS*, ed Gilbert Herdt, Clarendon Press, 1997, pp127–142

24. 'Men: the challenges of gender', Adriana Gómez, *Women's Health Journal*, January 1997, Latin American and Caribbean Women's Health Network, pp29–34
25. *New York Times Magazine*, 15 September 1996
26. Zimbabwean man quoted in 'Local voices', op cit [note 18] p38
27. *A Construção Cultural dos 'Meninos da Rua' no Rio do Janeiro: Implicações para a Prevenção de HIV/AIDS*, Patrick Larvie, Washington DC, AIDSCOM/AED, 1992, p40, quoted in *HIV and the Challenges Facing Men*, op cit [note 3] p7
28. "In a study of condom use among stable heterosexual couples [in Denmark] with a mean age of 30 years and with experience of condom use, 20 to 60 per cent of the men felt that the condom reduced the sensitivity of the penis." From 'The condom challenge', Bo Andreassan Rix, *Reproductive Health Matters*, May 1996, no 7, pp107–110
29. In San Francisco, however, where 'barebacking' has been well documented, HIV transmission rates appear to have fallen, for reasons that are not yet clear. *The Boston Globe*, 30 June 1998
30. Information from Dr Antonio Gerbase, World Health Organization, September 1998
31. For example, according to one study from Tanzania, 'being rich was a potential risk factor for [men] having multiple sexual partners': 'Determinants of high-risk sexual behaviour and condom use among adults in the Arusha region, Tanzania', Kagoma S Mnyika et al, *International Journal of STD and AIDS*, 1997, 8, pp176–183
32. *HIV and the Challenges Facing Men*, op cit [note 3] p5
33. ibid, p2

WOMEN MADE VULNERABLE

1. 'Local voices: what some Harare men say about preparation for sex', Sunanda Ray et al, *Reproductive Health Matters*, May 1996, 7, pp34–45
2. Dr Haroon Ahmed, former head of the department of psychiatry, Jinnah Hospital, quoted in 'The second sex', M Hanif, *Newsline*, Karachi, September 1992
3. 'Condom use in sexual exchange relationships among young single adults in Ghana', Augustine Ankomah, *AIDS Education and Prevention*, 1998, vol 10, no 4, pp303–316

4. 'Diffusion and focus in sexual networking: identifying partners and partners' partners', I.O. Orubuloye et al, in *Sexual Networking and AIDS in sub-Saharan Africa*, eds I.O. Orubuloye et al, Health Transition Centre/Australian National University, 1994, pp13–32

5. For example, 'Sexual behaviour in a fishing community on Lake Victoria, Uganda', Helen Pickering et al, *Health Transition Review*, 1997, vol 7, pp13–20

6. See for example 'Women's attitudes to men's sexual behaviour', O.B. Boroffice, *Health Transition Review*, supplement to vol 5, 1995, pp67–79

7. *Risks and Realities of Early Childbearing Worldwide*, Issues in Brief Paper, Alan Guttmacher Institute, New York and Washington, December 1996

8. 'Violence, rape and sexual coercion: everyday love in a South African township', K Wood and R Jewkes, in *Men and Masculinity*, ed C Sweetman, Oxfam, 1997

9. *The Guardian*, London, 4 November 1997, quoted in *Naz Ki Pukaar*, January 1998, no 20

10. Quoted in 'Studying domestic violence: perceptions of women in Chiapas, Mexico', N.M. Glantz and D.C. Halperin, *Reproductive Health Matters*, no 7, May 1996, pp122–127

11. Report in *The Asian Age*, London, 8 February 1997, quoted in *Naz Ki Pukaar*, July 1997, no 18

12. 'Sexuality and AIDS prevention among adolescents in Recife, Brazil', Ana Vasconcelos et al, International Center for Research on Women, June 1997

13. Quoted in 'The negotiating strategies determining coitus in stable heterosexual relationships', D Balmer et al, *Health Transition Review*, 1995, no 5, pp85–95

14. 'A challenge to the powerless woman', J Ross-Frankson, in *HIV and AIDS: The Global Inter-Connection*, ed E Reid, UNDP/Kumarian, 1995, p88

15. According to the *New York Times*, 23 April 1998, p1, and *The Economist*, 28 September 1996, girls are more successful than boys at school in the United States and many European countries; in the US four times as many boys as girls are diagnosed as emotionally disturbed, while twice as many boys as girls have learning difficulties.

16. 'Men, masculinity and "gender in development"', Andrea Cornwall, in *Men and Masculinity*, op cit [note 8]

17. 'Men, masculinities and the politics of development', Sarah C White, in *Men and Masculinity*, op cit [note 8]

18. *Pesquisa Sobre Saúde Reprodutiva e Sexualidade do Jovem, Rio de*

Janeiro, Curitiba, Recife 1989–1990, author unknown, Bemfam, Brazil, Centers for Disease Control, USA and US Department of Health Human Services, 1992, quoted in 'Adolescence: misunderstandings and hopes', María Helena Henriques-Mueller & João Yunes in *Gender, Women and Health in the Americas*, Pan American Health Organization, Scientific Publication no 541, 1993

19. 'Adolescence: misunderstandings and hopes', op cit [note 18]
20. 'Sexuality, condom use and gender norms among Brazilian teenagers', Vera Paiva, *Reproductive Health Matters*, November 1993, no 2, pp98–109
21. 'AIDS prevention through peer education for northern Thai single female and male migratory factory workers', Kathleen Cash and Wantana Busayawong, International Center for Research on Women, June 1997
22. *Risks and Realities of Early Childbearing Worldwide*, op cit [note 7]
23. *AIDS and the World II*, eds Jonathan M Mann & Daniel J.M. Tarantola, Oxford University Press, 1996, p465
24. As one example, in a three-country study in Africa in 1995 men were three times as likely to have knowledge of HIV/AIDS: 'Knowledge, opinions and attitudes towards AIDS in rural Africa (Senegal, Cameroon, Burundi)', M de Loenzien, *Sociétés d'Afrique & Sida* (in English), July 1996, no 13, pp11–13
25. 'Sexuality and AIDS prevention among adolescents in Recife, Brazil', op cit [note 12]
26. 'AIDS prevention through peer education for northern Thai single female and male migratory factory workers', op cit [note 21]
27. Story reported in 'Discourses of power and empowerment in the fight against HIV/AIDS in Africa', Carolyn Baylies & Janet Bujra, in *AIDS: Safety, Sexuality and Risk*, eds Peter Aggleton et al, Taylor & Francis, London, 1995
28. 'HIV prevalence risk in partner serodiscordance among pregnant women in Bangkok', Wimol Siriwasin et al, *Journal of the American Medical Association*, vol 280, no 1 pp49-54
29. See for example 'Discourses of power and empowerment in the fight against HIV/AIDS in Africa', op cit [note 27]
30. 'The negotiating strategies determining coitus in stable heterosexual relationships', op cit [note 13]
31. *HIV and AIDS: The Global Inter-Connection*, op cit [note 14] p147
32. 'Condom Use in Sexual Exchange Relationships Among Young Single Adults in Ghana', op cit [note 3]
33. Adapted from 'Tomorrow's era: gender, psychology and HIV infection', Lorraine Sherr, in *AIDS as a Gender Issue*, eds Lorraine Sherr et al, Taylor and Francis, London 1996

CHANGING MEN'S BEHAVIOUR

1. *Juntos, fuertes y orgullosos*, no 1, Guatemala City, October 1995
2. 'Abandoning self-defeating behaviors', Kim Best, *Network*, Family Health International, spring 1998, vol 18, no 3
3. 'Importance of education regarding sexual health with male members of the community in Pakistan', Francis Rufi Sardar et al, Abstract 34197, 12th World AIDS Conference, Geneva, 1998
4. 'Evolving a model for AIDS prevention education among underprivileged adolescent girls in urban India', A Bhende, *Women and AIDS Program Research Report Series*, Washington DC, 1995; quoted in *Vulnerability and Opportunity: Adolescents and HIV/AIDS in the Developing World*, Ellen Weiss et al, International Center for Research on Women, 1996, p9
5. This means fidelity to one's current long-term partner. When a relationship breaks up through death or separation, in any new relationship – even where both partners are faithful – condoms should be used until it can be proved that both partners are HIV-negative.
6. 'Changes in male sexual behaviour in response to the AIDS epidemic: evidence from a cohort study in urban Tanzania', Japheth Z.L. Ng'weshemi et al, *AIDS*, 1996, vol 10, pp1415–1420
7. *HIV and AIDS: The Global Inter-Connection*, ed Elizabeth Reid, UNDP/Kumarian, 1995, p141
8. 'Sexuality, condom use and gender norms among Brazilian teenagers', Vera Paiva, *Reproductive Health Matters*, November 1993, no 2, pp98–109
9. The statistics and much of the language in this paragraph come from 'Condom use increasing', William R Finger, Network, Family Health International, spring 1998, vol 18, no 3
10. 'Listening to khakis', Malcolm Gladwell, *New Yorker*, 28 July 1997
11. 'Male responsibility for reproductive health', Isaiah Ndong & William R Finger, *Network*, Family Health International, spring 1998, p29
12. POPLINE abstract: 'Africa takes a more male-friendly approach to family planning', D.O. Omuodo, *AIDS Analysis Africa*, December 1996, 6 (6), p14
13. 'Making space for young men in family planning clinics', John Seex, *Reproductive Health Matters*, May 1996, no 7
14. 'Male responsibility for reproductive health', op cit [note 11] p5
15. *Reaching Men Worldwide: Lessons Learned From Family Planning and Communication Projects, 1986–1996*, Johns Hopkins School of Public Health, Center for Communication Programs, Working Paper no 3, January 1997

16. Quoted in 'Condom use increasing', op cit [note 9]
17. *HIV & AIDS: The Global Inter-Connection*, op cit [note 7] p160
18. 'Norwegian gay men: reasons for the continued practice of unsafe sex', A Prieur, *AIDS Education and Prevention*, 1990, 2 (2), pp109–115; 'Promoting health', D Mechanic, *Society*, January/February 1990, pp16–22; both quoted in 'Migrancy, masculine identities and AIDS: the psychosocial context of HIV transmission on the South African gold mines', C Campbell, *Social Sciences Medicine*, 1997, vol 45 no 2, pp273–281
19. *Confronting AIDS: Public Priorities in a Global Epidemic*, World Bank/Oxford University Press, 1997
20. For example, 'AIDS stigma: a persistent social phenomenon in Mwanza, Tanzania', Soori Nnko, Abstract 34159, 12th World AIDS Conference, Geneva, 1998
21. *Community mobilization and AIDS*, UNAIDS technical update, April 1997
22. *Emerging Gay Identities in South Asia*, conference report, Humsafar Trust, Bombay, 1995

WHEN WOMEN SAY NO

1. 'La producción teórica sobre la masculinidad: nuevos aportes', Michael Kimmel, in *Fin de Siglo: Género y Cambio Civilizatorio*, Ediciones de las Mujeres, no 17, ISIS International, Santiago de Chile, 1992; quoted in 'Men: the challenges of gender', Adriana Gómez, *Women's Health Journal*, January 1997, Latin American and Caribbean Women's Health Network, pp29–34
2. Some of these statistics include physical and sexual violence by fathers in addition to husbands or other sexual partners.
3. Statistics from various sources quoted in *The State of Women in the World Atlas*, Joni Seager, Penguin Books USA, New York, 1997, pp26–27
4. ibid (Russian and US statistics)
5. Various studies, including *La violencia hacia la mujer como un problema de salud pública: la incidencia de la violencia doméstica en una microregión de la ciudad de Nezahualcóyotl*, Elizabeth Shrader Cox & Rosario Valdez, CECOVID, Mexico City, 1992
6. 'Violence, empowerment and women's health', Mayela García & Gloria Sayavedra, *The Right to Live Without Violence*, Latin American and Caribbean Women's Health Network, 1996
7. Information from the Procuraduría General de Justicia del Distrito Federal

8. Rural woman from Jalisco, quoted in 'Violence, empowerment and women's health', op cit [note 6]

9. Chichimeca woman from Guanajuato, ibid

10. 'The origins and control of domestic violence against women', Soledad Larrain & Teresa Rodríguez, in *Gender, Women and Health in the Americas*, Pan American Health Organization, 1993

11. *Sexism and the War System*, B Reardon, New York, 1985, quoted in 'The origins and control of domestic violence against women', op cit [note 10]

12. Urban woman from Jalisco, quoted in 'Violence, empowerment and women's health', op cit [note 6]

13. ibid

14. 'The origins and control of domestic violence against women', op cit [note 10]

15. ibid

16. 'La enfermedad se llama machismo', interview with Eduardo Liendro, *Revista Mujer Salud*, January 1997, pp45–52

17. Unpublished untitled paper, Carlos del Rio, director of CONASIDA, 12 June 1997

18. 'La enfermedad se llama machismo', op cit [note 16]

19. ibid

20. ibid

21. 'La imagen masculina del condón: una perspectiva de los varones jóvenes', José A Aguilar Gil & Luis Botello Lonngi (in preparation)

22. Quoted in *The Meanings of Macho: Being a Man in Mexico City*, Matthew C Gutmann, University of California, 1996, p116

23. 'Unequal status, unequal development: gender violence in Mexico', Patricia Duarte Sánchez & Gerardo González, in *Women against Violence: Breaking the Silence*, ed Ana Maria Brasileiro, UNIFEM, 1997

CHANGING TIMES?

1. 'Using rapid research to assist families affected by AIDS in Tanzania', S Hunter et al, *Health Transition Review*, 1997, vol 7 (supplement), pp393–420

2. 'Patterns of sexual behaviour in a rural population in North-Western Tanzania', Katua Munguti et al, *Social Sciences Medicine*, vol 44, no 10, pp1553–1561

3. 'Determinants of high-risk sexual behaviour and condom use among adults in the Arusha region, Tanzania', Kagoma S Mnyika et al, *International Journal of STD and AIDS*, 1997, vol 8, pp176–183; 'Patterns of sexual behaviour in a rural population in

North-Western Tanzania', op cit [note 2]. Note that the studies define 'casual sex' differently.

4. 'Patterns of sexual behaviour in a rural population in North-Western Tanzania', op cit [note 2]

5. 'Sexual behaviour survey in a rural area of northwest Tanzania', Elke Konings et al, *AIDS*, 1994, vol 8, no 7, pp987–993

6. However, one study points out that bar girls, who frequently have many sexual partners, tend to be better educated than the average woman: 'Sexual relationships, condom use and risk perception among female bar workers in north-west Tanzania', Z Mgalla & R Pool, *AIDS Care*, 1997, vol 9, no 4, pp407–416

7. Various studies reported in 'Determinants of high-risk sexual behaviour and condom use among adults in the Arusha region, Tanzania', op cit [note 3]

8. *Tanzanian school pupils and the discourse of sex*, Mwanza, TANESA Working Paper 3; referred to in 'Sexual relationships, condom use and risk perception among female bar workers in north-west Tanzania', op cit [note 6]

9. 'Determinants of high-risk sexual behaviour and condom use among adults in the Arusha region, Tanzania', op cit [note 3]

10. 'Changes in male sexual behaviour in response to the AIDS epidemic: evidence from a cohort study in urban Tanzania', Japheth Z.L. Ng'weshemi et al, *AIDS*, 1996, vol 10, no 12, pp1415–1420

11. 'Determinants of high-risk sexual behaviour and condom use among adults in the Arusha region, Tanzania', op cit [note 3]

12. ibid; also 'Patterns of sexual behaviour in a rural population in North-Western Tanzania', op cit [note 2]

13. 'Changes in male sexual behaviour in response to the AIDS epidemic', op cit [note 10]

14. 'Determinants of high-risk sexual behaviour and condom use among adults in the Arusha region, Tanzania', op cit [note 3]

THE SOUL IS WILLING

1. SEA-AIDS (internet) correspondence, 13 July 1998

2. Wassyla Tamzali, lawyer and specialist in women's rights at UNESCO, *New York Times*, 9 March 1998

3. *Bible:* Ephesians 5:22–23

4. *Koran:* Chapter 4, verse 34

5. *Bible:* Ephesians 5:25

6. *Koran:* Chapter 2, verse 187

7. *Bible:* I Corinthians 7:9

8. *Sahih Bukhari*: Volume 7, Book 62, Number 3
9. *Bible:* Proverbs 6:27–29
10. *Koran:* Chapter 17, verse 32; chapter 24, verse 2
11. *Koran:* Chapter 4, verse 3
12. *Bible:* Proverbs 5:3–11
13. *Bible:* Genesis 1:28

FROM BOYS TO MEN

1. Adapted from *Pesquisa Sobre Saúde Reprodutiva e Sexualidade do Jovem, Rio de Janeiro, Curitiba, Recife* 1989–1990, author unknown, Bemfam, Brazil, Centers for Disease Control, USA and US Department of Health Human Services, 1992, quoted in 'Adolescence: misunderstandings and hopes', María Helena Henriques-Mueller & João Yunes, in *Gender, Women and Health in the Americas*, Pan American Health Organization, Scientific Publication no 541, 1993

2. Studies referred to in *Vulnerability and Opportunity: Adolescents and HIV/AIDS in the Developing World*, Ellen Weiss et al, International Center for Research on Women, 1996, p6, indicate 32 percent of young women interviewed in Malawi and 9 percent in Brazil had intercourse before their first menstruation. One in four boys in a Nigerian study reported sexual experience before their 13th birthday: 'Sexual networking among youth in southwestern Nigeria', Donatus O Owuamanam, *Health Transition Review*, 1995, supplement to vol 5, pp57–66

3. *Impact of HIV and sexual health education on the sexual behaviour of young people*, UNAIDS, Geneva, 1997

4. For example, "over 75 percent of [Kenyan] children and adults were supportive of school-based family life education programs." Quote from 'Communicating about sex: adolescents and parents in Kenya', K Kiragu et al, AIDS/STD *Health Promotion Exchange*, 1996, no 3, pp11–13

5. 'Ugandan parents: agents for change in promoting the prevention of the sexual transmission of HIV', A Opio and E A Mortimer, *Understanding and Action, Newsletter of the Sociétés d'Afrique & Sida*, April 1996, no 12, and Abstract WeC262 of IX International Conference on STD and AIDS, Kampala, 1995. Note that the title does not reflect the content of the paper.

6. 'Training teachers to lead discussion groups on HIV/AIDS prevention with adolescents in Zimbabwe', Godfrey Welk et al, paper prepared for the International Center for Research on

Women, June 1997

7. 'Youth and sexual risk in Sri Lanka', K Tudor Silva et al, paper prepared for International Center for Research on Women, June 1997

8. 'The condom challenge', Bo Andreassen Rix in *Reproductive Health Matters*, May 1996, no 7, pp107–110

9. 'Adolescence: misunderstandings and hopes', op cit [note 1]

A DOUBLE LIFE

1. Records from cultures that no longer exist do not always mention sex between men, but there is sufficient evidence to indicate such behaviour is universal. For historical documentation there are many Asian and Arabic records, as well as *Patterns of Sexual Behavior*, C.S. Ford and F.A. Beach, London, Eyre and Spottiswoode, 1952. A more recent analysis of bisexual behaviour in 13 countries (in Europe, the Americas, Asia and Oceania) can be found in *Bisexualities and AIDS: International Perspectives*, ed Peter Aggleton, Taylor & Francis, London, 1996.

2. *India Visit 23rd November-28th December* 1996, Shivananda Khan, Naz Foundation, unpublished

3. 'Male bisexuality in Peru and the prevention of AIDS', Carlos F Cáceres, in *Bisexualities and AIDS*, op cit [note 1] pp136–147

4. *Cultural constructions of male sexualities in India*, Shivananda Khan, Naz Foundation, 1995

5. The word 'homosexual' as used in this chapter refers to desire, not behaviour, but it is often used by others to refer only to behaviour, or to desire and behaviour.

6. Statistics from Mexico, Norway and the United States quoted in 'La bisexualidad', José Antonio Izazola Licea, *Antología de la sexualidad humana*, vol III, M.A. Porrúa, 1994; Brazil in POPLINE summary of 'HIV infection and risk behaviors among male portworkers in Santos, Brazil', R Lacerda et al, *American Journal of Public Health*, August 1996, 86 (8), pp1158–60; Botswana in 'Notes on the socio-economic and cultural factors influencing the transmission of HIV in Botswana', D MacDonald, *Social Science Medicine*, 1996, vol 42, no 9, pp1325–1333; Peru in 'Sexual cultures and sexual health: young people and their current discourse, practice and risks regarding sexuality in Lima, Peru', Carlos F Caceres, *Abstracts of the XI International Conference on AIDS*, ThD440, Vancouver, 1996; Thailand (six percent) in 'The role of same-sex behavior in the HIV epidemic among northern Thai men', Chris Beyrer et al, Abstract 13136, 12th World AIDS

Conference, Geneva, 1998; Thailand (16 percent) in 'Socio-demographic correlates, HIV/AIDS-related cofactors and measures of same-sex sexual behaviour among Northern Thai male soldiers', Andrew S London et al, *Health Transition Review*, 1997, vol 7, pp33–60

7. *On the Margins*, Neil McKenna, Panos/Norwegian Red Cross, London, 1996
8. 'Emergence of gay identity and gay social movements in developing countries; the AIDS crisis as catalyst', Matthew W Roberts, *Alternatives*, 1995, vol 20, pp243–264
9. Wanjira Kiama is the pseudonym of a Kenyan journalist.
10. *Facing Mount Kenya*, J Kenyatta, Heinemann, London, 1979. In fact, as discussed later in this report, some African languages do have words to describe sex between men.
11. *Daily Nation*, Nairobi, 24 September 1995
12. *East African*, 22–29 October 1995

IN A COUNTRY WHERE NOBODY CARES

1. Estimates from Dr Don Des Jarlais, Chemical Dependency Institute, Beth Israel Medical Center, New York, April 1998
2. Dr Don Des Jarlais, April 1998
3. 'Women drug users and their partners', Hilary Klee, in *AIDS as a Gender Issue*, eds Lorraine Sher et al, Taylor and Francis, London, 1996, p166
4. To prevent transmission of HIV, hepatitis and other viruses, each injector should (a) use new sterile equipment, (b) boil all injecting equipment for a minimum of 10 minutes or (c) thoroughly immerse in full strength bleach for a minimum of 30 seconds. Washing in hot water is inadequate.
5. 'A model-based estimate of HIV infectivity via needle sharing', Edward H Kaplan & Robert Heimer, *Journal of Acquired Immune Deficiency Syndromes*, 1992, vol 5, pp1116–1118
6. 'Rising HIV infection rates in Ho Chi Minh City heralds emerging AIDS epidemic in Vietnam', Christina P Lindan et al, *AIDS*, 1997, 11 (supplement 1), ppS5–S13
7. 'Women drug users and their partners', op cit [note 3] pp163–176. However, some women who inject sell sex in order to buy drugs.
8. 'An international comparative study of HIV prevalence and risk behaviour among drug injectors in 13 cities', WHO Collaborative Study Group, Bulletin on Narcotics, 1993, vol 45, no 1, pp19–46
9. *The Social Impact of AIDS in the United States*, National Research

Council, National Academy Press, 1993, p272, quoted in *Sexual Ecology: AIDS and the destiny of gay men*, Gabriel Rotello, Dutton, New York, 1997, pp35–36

10. In 1973 the US federal prison system held 5,000 drug offenders; almost 11 times that number (54,000) were incarcerated 25 years later. In the same period the number of current users of illegal drugs in the United States was estimated to have fallen from 25 million in 1979 to 14 million in 1997.

11. 'Effectiveness of needle exchange programmes for prevention of HIV infection', S.F. Hurley et al, *Lancet*, 1997, vol 349 (9068), pp1797–1800

12. 'Epidemiology of HIV infection and AIDS in Thailand', B.G. Weniger et al, *AIDS*, 1991, vol 5 (supplement 2) pp71–85

13. 'AIDS epidemic in Kaliningrad', Pauli Leinikki, *Lancet*, 28 June 1997, vol 349, pp1914–1915

14. Information from Nikolai Nedzelsky, IMENA Project

15. Information from Dr Vadim Pokrovsky, director of the Ministry of Health Anti-AIDS Prevention Programme

16. *Durex Global Sex Survey* 1997

17. *AIDS Weekly Plus*, 30 June 1997

18. Research in New York indicates that two percent of HIV-negative injecting drug users die each year, in comparison with four to five percent of HIV-positive injectors (information from Dr Don Des Jarlais). If 30 percent of a group of drug users in New York are HIV-positive, a rough interpretation of these figures suggests that half of the whole group will live for more than 20 years and slightly fewer than one in four of those who die will do so from HIV-related causes.

19. *Los Angeles Times*, 5 November 1997

20. ibid

21. ibid

22. ibid

HELL ON EARTH

1. '(Ir)relevance of condoms in prisons', Hernán Reyes, International Committee of the Red Cross, presentation at CHS conference in Sydney, November 1997

2. *Prisons and AIDS: UNAIDS Point of View*, UNAIDS Best Practice Collection, April 1997

3. Sexual contact also takes place in female prisons, but the risks of HIV transmission in such a situation are low.

4. *Prisons and AIDS*, op cit [note 2]
5. 'Sexual networking, STDs and HIV/AIDS in four urban gaols in Nigeria', I.O. Orubuloye et al, *Health Transition Review*, 1995, supplement to vol 5, 123–129
6. '(Ir)relevance of condoms in prisons', op cit [note 1]
7. *Prisons and AIDS*, op cit [note 2]
8. ibid
9. In a very few countries, such as the Netherlands, prison authorities are required by law to provide condoms free of charge to prisoners. In some prisons a laissez-faire policy has been adopted where condoms are provided by the medical service although not officially approved by the prison authorities. (Information adapted from '(Ir)relevance of condoms in prisons', op cit [note 1])
10. '(Ir)relevance of condoms in prisons', op cit [note 1]
11. Most transvestites in Brazil (*travestis*), as in some other countries, are men who live most or all of their lives as women. Many take hormones to enhance their breasts but do not have surgery to replace their genital organs. Transsexuals wish to have surgery but may live as women for many years before doing so.
12. 'closet homosexuals': men who prefer not to admit in public their sexual preference for other men
13. This section was adapted, with kind permission, from 'Bisexual communities and cultures in Costa Rica', Jacobo Schifter et al, in *Bisexualities and AIDS: International Perspectives*, ed Peter Aggleton, Taylor & Francis, London, 1996.

ACROSS THE BORDER

1. The language in this paragraph, and many of the points in this section, have been adapted from *HIV/AIDS Strategy in Latin America and Africa: Military and Civil-Military Policies and Issues*, ed Sven Groennings, Civil Military Alliance to Combat HIV and AIDS, Occasional Paper no 1, April 1997.
2. *AIDS and the Military*: UNAIDS Point of View, May 1998
3. Military statistics, except Thailand, from *HIV/AIDS Strategy in Latin America and Africa*, op cit [note 1]; Thai military statistics from Stuart Kingma, co-director Civil-Military Alliance to Combat HIV and AIDS; adult population statistics from UNAIDS, December 1997
4. *HIV/AIDS Strategy in Latin America and Africa*, op cit [note 1]
5. *Understanding Prevention: A Primary Mission for Military Medical Services*, Stuart Kingma, Civil Military Alliance Newsletter, July 1997, vol 3, no 3

6. 'Socio-demographic correlates, HIV/AIDS-related cofactors, and measures of same-sex sexual behaviour among Northern Thai male soldiers', Andrew S London et al, *Health Transition Review*, 1997, vol 7, pp33–60

7. 'Disintegration conflicts and the restructuring of masculinity', Judith Large, in *Gender and Development*, June 1997, vol 5, no 2, pp23–30; this study refers to other sources, including *Study on Child Soldiers*, R Brett, Quaker United Nations Office, Geneva, 1996, for higher numbers of boy soldiers compared with girl soldiers; and *Child Soldiers: the role of children in armed conflicts*, Clarendon Press, Oxford, n.d.

8. Figure from United Nations High Commissioner for Refugees (UNHCR)

9. For a more extensive analysis of the impact of conflict on women, see *Arms to Fight, Arms to Protect*, ed Olivia Bennett, Panos, London, 1995

10. Rape of men in Croatia was reported in *The Guardian*, London, 29 July 1996, according to 'Disintegration conflicts and the restructuring of masculinity', op cit [note 7]

11. *The State of Women in the World Atlas*, Joni Seagar, Penguin Books USA, New York, 1997

12. *WorldAIDS,* March 1995, p3

13. *Times of India*, 28 February 1997, quoted in *Naz Ki Pukaar*, July 1997, no 18, p14

14. *HIV/AIDS Strategy in Latin America and Africa*, op cit [note 1] p35

15. ibid, p70

To Mark My Time on Earth

1. 'Infancy and early childhood: cross-cultural codes 2', H Barry & L M Paxson, *Ethnology*, 1971, 10, pp466–508, quoted in 'Fathers as parenting partners', Patrice L Engle & Ann Leonard, *Families in Focus: New Perspectives on Mothers, Fathers and Children*, J Bruce et al, Population Council, New York, 1995, pp49–69

2. *HIV and AIDS: The Global Inter-Connection*, ed Elizabeth Reid, UNDP/Kumarian, New York, 1995, p161

3. 'The role of men in families: achieving gender equity and supporting children', Patrice L Engle, in *Men and Masculinity*, ed C Sweetman, Oxfam, 1997, pp31–40

4. The points in this paragraph come from various papers cited in 'The role of men in families', op cit [note 3]; also papers cited in *Sex on the Brain*, Deborah Blum, Viking, New York, 1997, pp123–125.

5. The points and quotes in this paragraph come from 'Progenitors changing response to teenage pregnancy', Irma Palma and Cecilia Quilodrán, *Women's Health Journal*, January 1997, Latin American and Caribbean Women's Health Network, pp43–46

6. *HIV and AIDS: The Global Inter-Connection*, op cit [note 2] p114

7. Although this option is increasingly available in the developing world, most pregnant women still do not have access to the drug.

8. See for example 'Using rapid research to develop a national strategy to assist families affected by AIDS in Tanzania', S Hunter et al, *Health Transition Review*, 1997, vol 7, (supplement), pp393–420, and references quoted therein

9. 'Masculinity and the male role model in sexual health', Bonnie Shepherd, *Planned Parenthood Challenges*, 1996, no 2, pp11–14

10. All figures except the last from *SIDA en Côte d'Ivoire*, December 1997, Programme National de Lutte contre le SIDA, les MST et la Tuberculose, Ministry of Health, Abidjan. Figure of 15,000 children born with HIV based on estimate of 700,000 births a year, nine percent of pregnant women being HIV-positive and 25 percent mother-to-child transmission rates.

11. All figures in this paragraph from a 1992 report to WHO/GPA authored by Séri Dedy & Gozé Tapé

12. ibid

13. Information from Dr Youdjé Gnonsoa-Ateby, PSI

14. *The needs of families affected by HIV/AIDS in Cote d'Ivoire and the institutional responses to assist them*, Melissa Root, unpublished paper, 1998

15. ibid

16. *SIDA en Côte d'Ivoire*, op cit [note 10]

PANOS (LONDON)

The Panos Institute in London exists to stimulate debate on global environment and development issues. Panos does not advocate solutions but provides information, presenting different arguments and perspectives to enable people to form their own opinions and find their own solutions.

Founded in 1986, the Panos Institute raises awareness of neglected or poorly understood issues and communicates the concerns of marginalised sectors of society. Panos promotes the plurality and diversity of the media by working with community and information organisations worldwide and supporting their communication activities through such means as newspapers, local language features services, radio programmes, investigative studies and oral testimony collection.

Panos supports journalists in the developing world in their reporting of local environment, health, gender, media and development concerns, through commissioning, workshops, seminars and other initiatives. Panos considers the process of gathering and sharing information to be as important as the outcome; people learn from the experience and attitudes can change along the way.

As well as catalysing debate on a national and regional level, Panos works to ensure that perspectives from developing countries reach the Northern public through the media, thus increasing the exchange of ideas and experience between developing countries and the industrialised world.

Panos offices exist in a number of countries. Panos London has been instrumental in establishing offices in Addis Ababa, Kathmandu and Lusaka, which work in Eastern Africa, South Asia and Southern Africa respectively.

THE PANOS AIDS PROGRAMME

The Panos AIDS Programme was established with the founding of Panos in 1986. The programme aims to provide accurate and relevant information on the extent, causes and implications of the global HIV/AIDS epidemic, and to stimulate public and policy debate on the response. Its primary partners are the media in the developing world, but the programme also works on an occasional basis with non-governmental and government organisations, as well as other institutions and individuals.

The programme's first publication, *AIDS and the Third World* (1986), was instrumental in alerting the media, governments, non-governmental organisations, medical staff and others around the world to the growing threat of the HIV/AIDS epidemic. Since then, Panos has provided extensive coverage and analysis of the epidemic, through publications and sponsorship of workshops, seminars and research.

The programme has also worked with Panos South Asia and Panos Washington, which provides information on HIV/AIDS in Spanish for Latin America.

In 1996-1998 Panos AIDS Features, Briefings and Information Sheets were circulated worldwide. *On the Margins* by Neil McKenna (1996) raised awareness of the relationship between HIV and sex between men in the developing world. Both that title and *The Silent Epidemic* (forthcoming) - a shorter, updated summary - are available free of charge in the developing world and for sale in industrialised countries.

In 1999-2000 the AIDS Programme will continue to support meetings, research and publication on the topic of AIDS and Men as experienced in different communities across the world. The programme will also focus on the implications of HIV testing, counselling and treatment.

AIDS AND MEN

Taking Risks or
Taking Responsibility?

edited with an introduction by

Martin Foreman

PANOS/Zed Books

Published by The Panos Institute and Zed Books

The Panos Institute
9 White Lion Street
London N1 9PD, UK
Tel: +44 (0)171 278 1111
E-mail: panos@panoslondon.org.uk
Web site: http://www.oneworld.org/panos

Zed Books Ltd
7 Cynthia Street
London N1 9JF
Tel: + 44 (0) 171 837 4014
E-mail: sales@zedbooks.demon.co.uk
Web site: http://www.zedbooks.demon.co.uk

Distributed exclusively in the USA by
St Martin's Press Inc
175 Fifth Avenue, New York
NY 10010, USA

British Library Cataloguing in Publication Data.
A catalogue record for this book is available from the British Library
IBSN 1870670 40X pb
    185649 7445 hb

Extracts may be freely reproduced by the press or non-profit organisations, with acknowledgement. Panos would appreciate clippings of published materials based on *AIDS and Men: Taking Risks or Taking Responsibility?*

Funding for the AIDS and Men programme was provided by the Norwegian Red Cross, the Swiss Agency for Development and Cooperation and the Swedish International Development Cooperation Agency. The Panos AIDS Programme also receives regular financial support from the Royal Danish Ministry of Foreign Affairs and the Ford Foundation. No opinions expressed in this document should be taken to represent the views of any funding agency or reviewer. Signed articles do not necessarily reflect the views of Panos or any of its funding agencies.

The introductory chapters and the introductions to each country report were written by Martin Foreman, Director of the Panos AIDS Programme.

Some of the names of people interviewed in the country reports have been changed to protect their identities.

Additional research: Jill Shipway
Managing editors: Heather Budge-Reid and James Deane
Final text editing: Daniel Nelson and John Hilary
Design and production: Sally O'Leary
Printed: Cambrian Printers, Aberyswyth
Front cover picture: Heldur Netocny/Panos Pictures